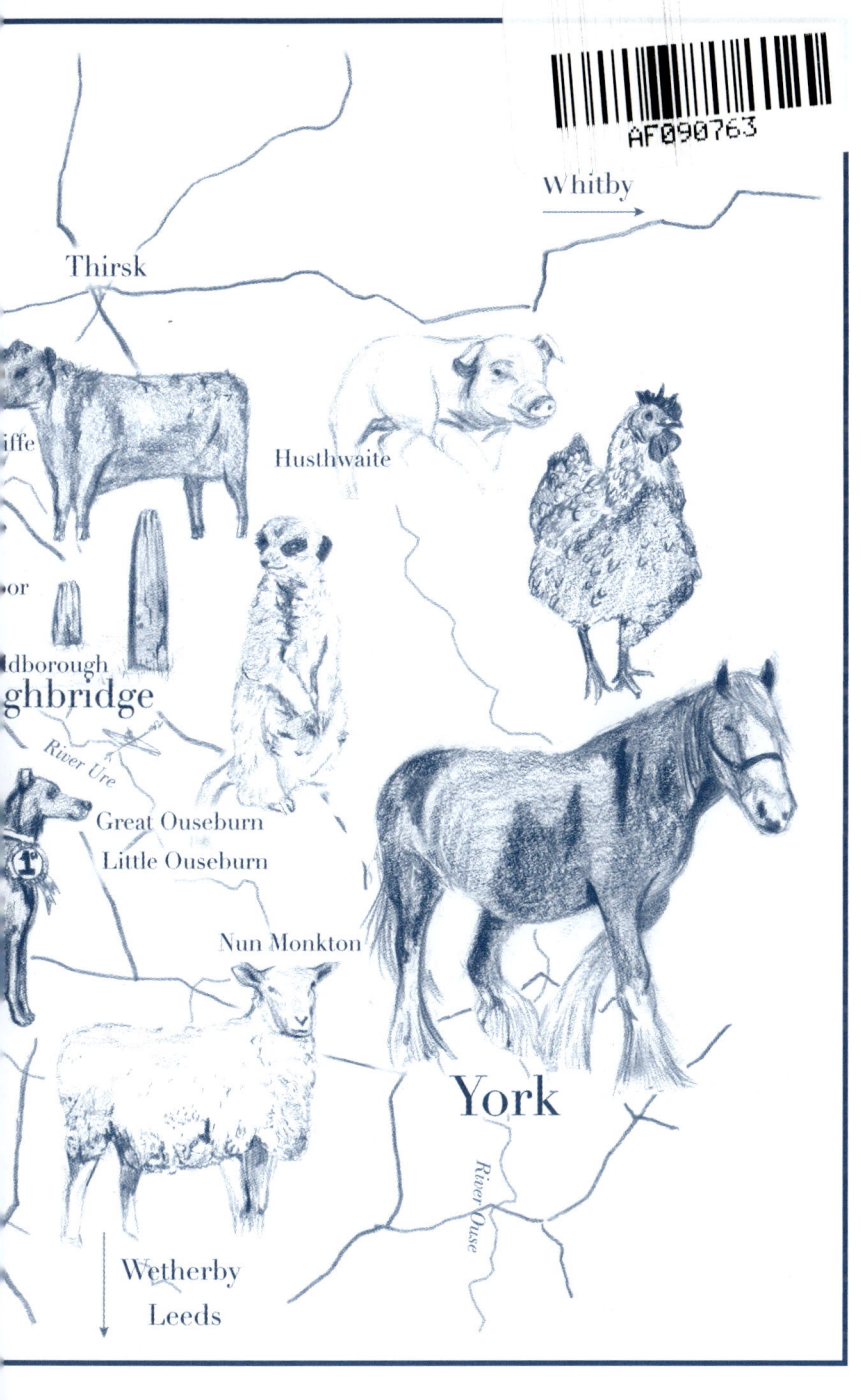

A YORKSHIRE VET
back to
HERRIOT COUNTRY

JULIAN NORTON

GREAT *N*ORTHERN

Great Northern Books Limited
PO Box 1380, Bradford, BD5 5FB
www.greatnorthernbooks.co.uk

© Julian Norton 2025

Every effort has been made to acknowledge correctly and contact the copyright holders of material in this book. Great Northern Books Limited apologises for any unintentional errors or omissions, which should be notified to the publisher.

All rights reserved. No part of this book may be reproduced in any form or by any means without permission in writing from the publisher, except by a reviewer who may quote brief passages in a review.

ISBN: 978-1-914227-81-3

Design and layout: David Burrill
Front cover image: Lucy Pittaway www.lucypittaway.co.uk
Back cover image: Jack Norton

CIP Data
A catalogue for this book is available from the British Library

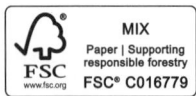

Contents

Foreword 5
Puppy Party, Diarrhoea and Lazy Science 7
Dogs Who Look Like Their Owners 9
In Praise of Dogs 11
Mini the Guinea 13
Canine Altruism 15
CUMC 17
Swan Rescue! 19
Springtime 21
Stary Smokovec 23
Turn-Out Time 25
Restricted Access 27
Boris Has Been Helpful 29
Gerald, Thomas and Christopher 31
Sponge Bob; Square Stomach 33
Stories from Scotland (1) 35
Stories from Scotland (2) 37
Oystercatcher 39
Benzene Ring 41
Dog Treats 43
Getting Old? 45
Yew Turn 47
Birthday Ziggy 49
Sheep on Hay Bales 51
Nice People 54
Dressing Gowns 56
Hamster in Space! 58
Collapsed Lungs 60
She's Electric 62
Swiss Epic 64
Wild Animal Rescue 67
Swallows on the Wire 69
Smelly Cat 71
RDA 73
Ambushed by a Cat 75
Head in a Watering Can 77
Well Oiled 79

Skippy	81
Goodbye Brucella, Hello Other Diseases	83
Encouraging Kids to Read	85
Dogs on Tables?	87
Emmy in the Wars	89
Trainees	91
A Herriot Trainee	93
Conference Season	95
Toilet Dog	97
Six Dinner Sid? No Dinners Brian	99
Jamie and the Magic Torch?	101
I Am the Walrus	103
Five Poorly Mice	105
Wimba Way!	107
Special Patients	109
Vets in the Community	111
Shagging in the Pub	114
Taxi Deliveroo	116
Boston, Lincs	118
Henges	120
Crufts	122
Opening Libraries	124
Libraries (2)	126
Lambing Time	128
Opening the Fridge	130
Complicated Surgery	132
Ferret Castration; Ferret Vasectomy	134
Naughty Gus	136
Race Mode	138
Catching Up	140
Death by Mince Pie	142
Jess and the Magic Spell	144
Melancholy; Vultures	146
Vultures	148
Flower Farm and Happy Farm	150
Henley Royal Regatta	152
Polish Thesis, Wittgenstein and Dogs in Prams	155
Alpacas	157
Acknowledgements	159

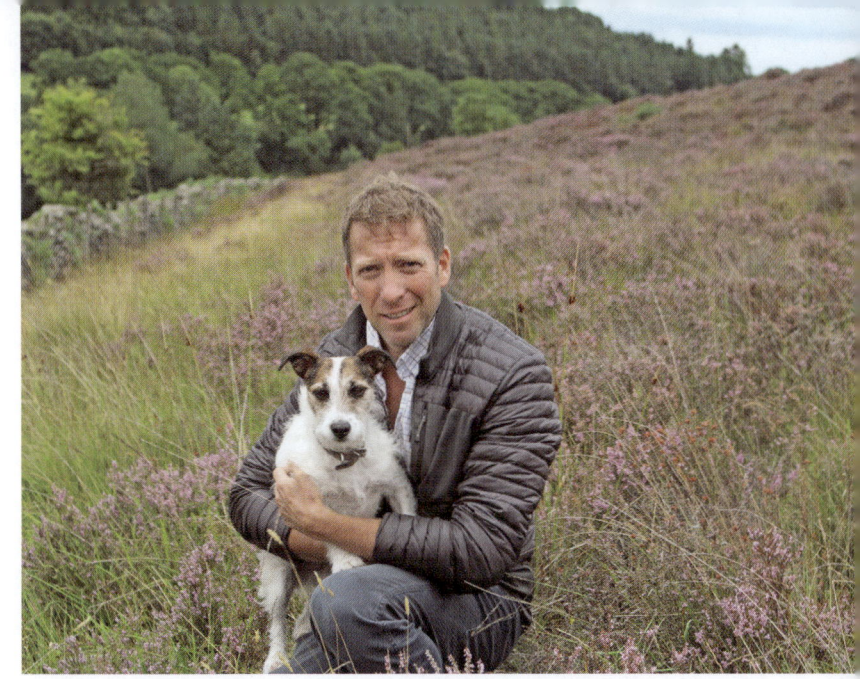

Foreword

This, my latest "diary" style book in the series, is a collection of stories from my veterinary life. These anecdotes come from the time just after Anne, Isabella and I had opened our new practice, Thirsk Veterinary Centre. A bit like Sandbeck, down the road in Wetherby – which is just over a year its senior and functions like an older sibling to the new practice – its inception came about through good fortune and lucky circumstance. Anne and Isabella had worked together for several years and ideas were starting to develop about striking out on their own. They were both putting in long and hard hours in a practice where the boss was rarely around. Surely, they could do it themselves? I suggested the idea of opening a practice in Thirsk. We could run it as a sister practice to Sandbeck, sharing the same ethos, systems, logos, some equipment and staff (which would be mainly me). We could reduce the risk and the stress of an otherwise daunting venture. Ever since I'd been ousted from veterinary practice in my home town, back in December 2017, I'd had a feeling that there was unfinished veterinary business in Thirsk with its historic links to James Herriot. On dog walks and when shopping in town, people would come up and ask on a regular basis, "When are you going to set up here?"

I'd shrug and give a non-committal answer. Besides, I was actually enjoying working away from my own front door. Given my circumstances and involvement in *The Yorkshire Vet*, it provided a small screen of anonymity, which was both welcome and unusual. But some words from the corporate boss who bought Skeldale kept haunting me. He was confident his takeover of, arguably, the most historic veterinary practice in the world would be a success and that I, a minor nuisance, who had failed to toe the line and resisted with all my might throughout, would present no problems for the gargantuan expansion of his growing conglomerate. "We are not worried, Julian. Within a couple of years, everyone in Thirsk will have forgotten who you are."

No doubt, after many acquisitions and ultimately one big sale, as he relaxes in his chateau or on his yacht, *he* has totally forgotten about me; I'm not so sure the same is true for some of my old friends, clients and patients.

So, we secured a brilliant location, on the site of Thirsk Rural Business Centre, which was fitting, as it placed us right back at the epicentre of the rural community, with good access and endless parking. There was even an uninterrupted view of the white stone cliff and Sutton Bank. In March 2021, independent veterinary practice returned to Herriot's home town. We opened our doors with some trepidation. Would people come? Would the phone ring? Did we have sufficient staff; or were there too many?

We need not have worried. It was good to be back in Herriot Country!

Puppy Party, Diarrhoea and Lazy Science

It was chaos last Saturday. Morning surgery was full, with plenty of extras to slot in. Most of these seemed to be cases of gastroenteritis, which veterinary surgeons all over the country, and particularly across Yorkshire, have been busy with for the last few weeks. Media articles proclaimed the cause to be "something on the beach". Apparently, the finger of suspicion pointed towards mounds of dead crabs. However, this limited journalistic investigation failed to identify the fact that many cases of the mystery illness were popping up in dogs who lived inland and had not visited a beach for months, let alone encountered crustaceans. A quick count-up showed that our practice in Wetherby had seen thirty cases of vomiting and diarrhoea in three days. At Thirsk, too, ten per day seemed to be the average. But the dramatic headlines were bereft of accurate detail or facts, which, sadly, is something to which we are all now accustomed. Maybe it was the "deadly E. coli virus" I read somewhere. Well, E. coli, as every GCSE scientist knows, is a bacteria and NOT a virus and the two organisms are very different. In my view, speculative reporting and a lazy approach to science is as dangerous as any diarrhoea-inducing virus (or bacteria).

But back to the diarrhoea dogs. The pattern seemed the same – vomiting two or three times at the outset, followed by nasty diarrhoea with a reduced appetite and loss of *joie de vivre*. Most dogs I've seen, to be fair, have not been extremely ill. Dehydration seems to have been relatively mild and the dogs have responded well to treatment. A few have needed more intensive care, such as intravenous fluids and an overnight stay. But one poor lady, exasperated and short of sleep with three spaniels all suffering, looked as strained as the dogs' bowels. As they wagged their way into my consulting room, one immediately produced a copious and unhealthy sample right in the middle of my consulting room floor.

"My goodness," I said. "I bet your kitchen is a big mess?"

"Well, the kitchen's not too bad," she sighed. "The worst thing is that they all sleep in the bedroom with me."

As I drew up three syringes of medication, I hoped my treatment would produce rapid results … and I tried not to picture the scene *chez spaniels*.

The cause, of course, is unlikely to be poisonous crabs, washed up onto Britain's beaches, having succumbed to their own deadly virus or bacteria. The British Small Animal Veterinary Association is busy compiling data on the outbreak, but the ubiquitous and seasonal build-up of pathogens, both specific and non-specific, that accumulate in the sticky mud across the country every winter, especially when it's been mild, without hard frosts to contain the bugs, is probably the culprit. Dogs live near the ground. They lick all sorts of tasty stuff on the pavements, they lick themselves in all sorts of grubby places and their natural greeting is to sniff another dog's bottom. Some eat cat poo. Others delight in rabbit, horse or sheep faeces. And they definitely do not wash their paws for twenty seconds while singing happy birthday, nor use hand sanitiser after being outside. With habits like that, is there any wonder they get vomiting and diarrhoea?

But by lunchtime on Saturday, all the dogs with diarrhoea had gone home and all parts of the waiting room had been scrubbed and thoroughly disinfected. More chaos was about to kick off. We were ready to host our first post-Covid puppy party! We all hoped the puppies could hold onto their bowels, because we'd had enough poo for one day!

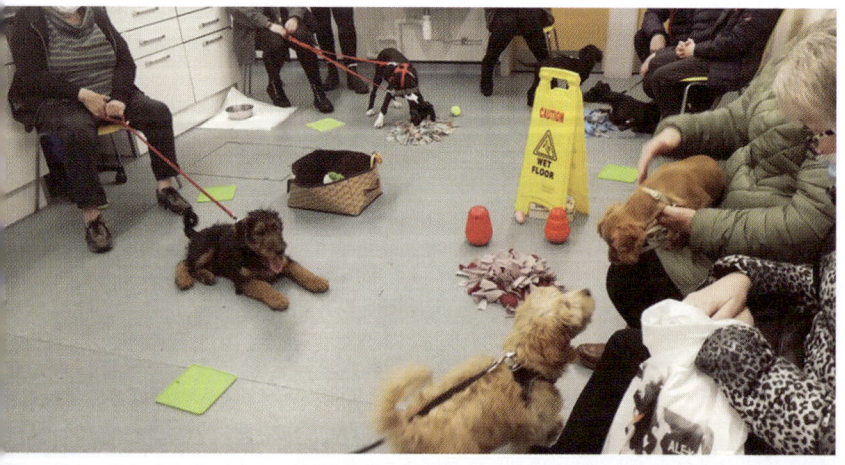

Dogs Who Look Like Their Owners

I've touched on the fascinating topic of "dogs who look like people" before. The last time, it was with reference to a dog who looked just like, and was named after, a character in a film. The mop-headed poodle-cross was called Bhodi, after the surf-dude character played by the late and great Patrick Swayze in the film *Point Break*. The similarity was striking. I don't usually re-visit topics in this column, as there is always a plentiful supply of stories from the veterinary and animal world, but a recent evening event reminded me of this amusing subject, so I thought I could break my habit, just this once.

I was at the excellent Arts Centre in Pocklington, sitting on a chair on stage, in conversation with my friend Adam. This was one of the first of these events I'd done for some time, as the pandemic had put a stop to evenings at the theatre. Now, as life finally opened back up to a semblance of normality, I lugged a box of my books into the foyer, hoping I'd sell a few at the interval. I'd optimistically purchased a mountain of books pre-Covid, and most of them were still sitting, stoically, in boxes piled high in the spare bedroom, gathering dust. Their presence acted as an irksome reminder of my, often misplaced, optimism. Two years ago, I optimistically predicted this new virus would be a flash in the pan and over by summer. I was very wrong. Nonetheless, if the audience was a reasonable size, I hoped I stood a chance of getting rid of a few dozen in Pocklington that evening.

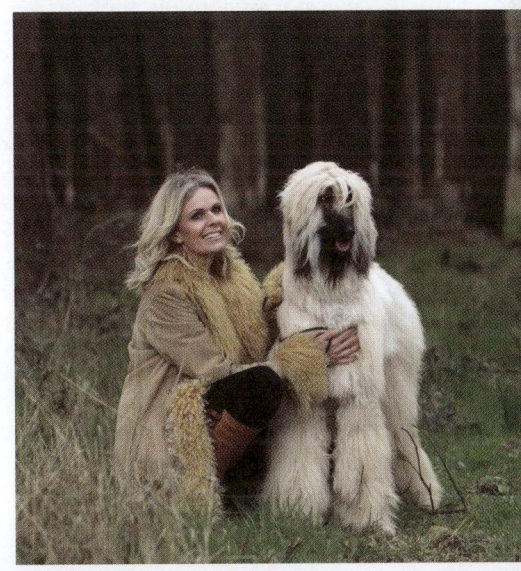

The venue was impressive,

situated in the centre of the high street in "Pock". I'd arrived in good time and found a convenient place to park right outside (so carrying books was easy). I met Adam, who lived just down the road, and we lurked in the green room beforehand.

As we ran through some last-minute ideas for topics to talk about, I glanced at the pictures of previous performers in this lovely little venue. John Bishop had sold out on two consecutive nights. Ade Edmonson, from *The Young Ones*, and Phill Jupitus were there too. All available wall space was covered in posters. It sent my stomach into knots, because this is still uncomfortable territory for me. Toyah Willcox was coming soon too.

The first half went well and we reconvened during the interval to chat about the next part, which would mainly consist of questions from the audience, some collected in advance. Adam usually keeps these questions to himself but gave me advanced warning of one in particular. "Is it true that owners very often look exactly like their dogs?"

The topic was discussed in some detail during the second half. I concurred that it was a thing, related the story of Bhodi and described the often-seen pairing of a body builder with a bulldog. After other examples, I rounded off the discussion by alluding to the classic owner/dog look-a-like combo that I had not yet encountered; that of a beautiful blonde owning an Afghan hound, with matching flowing golden locks.

Later that week, an email arrived at my practice, from a lady who had been a member of the audience on that evening. She was too shy to put up her hand on the night, but attached to the email was a photograph.

"This is a photo of my dog groomer and her hound," it said. "I hope you like it!"

In Praise of Dogs

I was surprised to read a recent description of dogs as "the plague" and their owners as selfish, arrogant and self-important. Out on my morning dog walk, I encountered quite a few dogs – none of them acting in a plague-like fashion – and their owners, none of whom appeared selfish, arrogant or self-important. In fact, everyone was very friendly. One older chap, with blue ears and a big red nose, had clearly misjudged the temperature and the direction from which the wind was blowing. "I wish I'd put my hat on," he complained, whilst grinning widely. There were other conversations, too, mostly in praise of the glorious sunshine, with the usual undertones of despondency about the mud.

"Well, it is March," I replied, in defence (of the mud).

On a sunny weekend morning, the patch of publicly owned open pasture near where we live is a happy place. It is grazed by a free-roaming and melancholic herd of young stirks, in various shades of brown. On a warm day in summer, they stand in the beck to cool their feet, alongside the brave youth of Thirsk who can often be found paddling and swimming. In March, the beck is too cold and deep for any of this, so the cattle wander, grazing on the last of the winter grass. One was trundling along the riverside path and came to investigate Emmy. She wasn't on a lead (because clinging onto a dog on a lead in the face of oncoming cattle is a sure-fire way of getting badly or even fatally injured) but she wasn't interested in a bullock, and skipped on, intent on looking for discarded tennis balls. Later, we found another herd member investigating a bush. The springer spaniel which rushed past, replete with new hair-cut and bright pink rubber ball, was too preoccupied to notice. Bill, in his eighties, shuffled along after his "new" terrier. He has recently lost both his wife and his geriatric Labrador, but the roly-poly little Jack Russell that he had rescued had given him a reason to get back out in the fresh air. In the distance, on the far side of a large puddle, a gang of dogs were having a great time while their owners enjoyed a chat. Even the elderly Shih Tzu, with his tongue hanging out of the front of his toothless mouth, was having fun. His old legs were too short to keep up with the youngsters, but he didn't seem to mind. Meanwhile, in the still-bare trees, birds sang, declaring that spring was on its way. It was a scene of human and animal amity – a tonic, especially at a time of global aggression, hostility and unpleasantness.

But animal amity was of no great surprise to me. The human/canine bond is strong. It is one that brings solace, support and mutual benefit and dates back through antiquity. A grave has been discovered in Jordan, dating back 16,500 years, in which a man was buried with his dog. This was around the time sapiens settled in the Americas and three millennia before the agricultural revolution (in which canines, incidentally, formed an integral part).

Later, back in front of my computer, I opened an email from the owners of a dog called "Bear". It went like this:

Dear Julian, Helen and Ed,

We just wanted to say Thank you for the care you gave to our special Bear. From Julian's diagnosis to the way the whole of Bear's end of life was dealt with by Ed was above and beyond and meant the world to all of us. Thank you for your empathy, your honesty and the caring nature of the whole team. Thank you from the bottom of our hearts.

Not selfish, not arrogant, not self-important.

Mini the Guinea

Guinea pigs are great. They have huge personalities and develop interesting inter-pig relationships, as well as amusing pig–human interactions. I used to sit with a cup of tea, after a busy day at work, with our two, Sparkle and Shine. I'd take them a stick of celery or a bunch of parsley and relate the woes and joys of my day. They both munched furiously and listened intently. At least I think they did. I'm pretty sure the squeaks and snuffles confirmed their agreement. I can say with confidence that they are excellent pets for small children and adults alike.

But when they go wrong, an ill guinea pig is an irksome challenge for any vet. They are difficult to examine and hard to investigate. Blood samples are challenging – if not impossible – to collect and interpret. X-rays can be useful up to a point (mainly to detect bladder stones) but it's hard to keep a "cavy" stationary for the X-ray exposure. Sedation or general anaesthesia is not so straightforward either. So, vets have to use a good dose of instinct and initiative to deal with sick pigs.

Mini had been a maxi challenge from the start. Initially, the cute and bristly guinea pig had shown very vague signs. She had a poor appetite and was reluctant to eat, but there were no other signs of illness. I examined her all over and checked her teeth – a common cause of GP malaise – but they were not too bad. Precautionary radiographs did not reveal anything obvious, leaving us at something of a diagnostic dead end. Luckily, before long, a clue appeared. Mini developed a discharge. A course of antibiotics was called for, which cleared up the nasty pus and her appetite returned. But as soon as the drugs finished, Mini relapsed, and it became clear that something more major needed to be done.

"I think we'll need to operate," I declared, outwardly confident but inwardly worried. My ambitious plan was to spay her, removing what was clearly a problematic uterus. The last time I'd done this to a guinea pig, the patient had huge, cystic ovaries and it was very tense, particularly as the patient belonged to a primary school. There was not one, but thirty worried children on operation day. Luckily, it was all fine and afterwards I was even invited to the school, where the pig was carried in for my inspection, sitting on a velvet cushion! I hoped Mini's surgery would be as smooth.

The day of Mini's surgery arrived and I promised to call as soon as I'd finished, whether with good news or bad. Everyone was anxious – owner, vet, and surgical nurse Lucy who had the unenviable job of maintaining a smooth anaesthetic.

Of course, she's very good and I shouldn't have been surprised that the GA and surgery went to plan. As she recovered, I peered at Mini's ovaries and uterus which lay on the surgical drape. They looked surprisingly normal. I picked up the scalpel again and sliced into one floppy tube. Its contents explained everything. A piece of hay, less than one centimetre long, was lodged high up in the uterus, almost at the fallopian tube. I have never seen anything like this before. The spikey foreign body must have worked its way upwards and was the obvious cause of her illness. It didn't seem huge, but a quick calculation of relative scale confirmed that it would be approximately equivalent to a cocktail stick stuck in a Jack Russell! More than enough to cause a problem. I crossed my fingers that the removal of Mini's mini fragment of hay would return her to maximum health!

Canine Altruism

Arianna was not feeling very grand. In fact, she was very poorly, suffering from a severe form of anaemia. Her immune system had gone wonky so that, rather than attacking the various viruses and bacteria that challenge a dog's body, it was aiming its forces against its own red blood cells. The result was a condition called Immune-mediated Haemolytic Anaemia. Frequently, this condition responds well to medication, but for Arianna, this was not the case. Both her blood count and chances of survival were fading rapidly. The only solution was to perform a blood transfusion. In a veterinary practice, this always causes excitement. It is not something we do very often, is usually very urgent and, in most cases, needs an emergency donor. An excellent service called the Pet Blood Bank has been developed over recent years, to coordinate and help to distribute bags of life-saving blood, but late on a Friday night, it's more often a frantic round of phone calls to the benevolent owners of benign large breed dogs that's required.

"Hello, it's Julian from the vet's. I'm sorry to disturb you on an evening, but I wondered if your lovely dog Larry would like to help save another dog's life," I spluttered down the telephone, or words to that effect. Of course, I went on the explain the situation in more detail, but I hoped my opening gambit would appeal to an altruistic owner, even though the chunky Labrador might not know anything about altruism.

"And there are ad lib biscuits and treats for the duration of the procedure, as well as afterwards," I added. There was mumbling at the other end of the phone, obviously Larry's owner was putting the question to Larry. Not only was he free, but he would definitely like to help save a life. And he would like free biscuits. He was there, ready, waiting and wagging outside the front door of the practice when the first staff arrived at eight the next morning. Arianna, who had been resting quietly and pallidly overnight, lifted her floppy head and attempted an appreciative wag. Larry was lined up and everything was ready. Dogs have a similar blood arrangement to humans, although the "Dog Erythrocyte Antigens" (DEAs) do not have corresponding auto-antibodies, as we humans do (that sounds complicated, and it is a bit). Basically, it means that it is safe to perform one blood transfusion without doing a cross match. That said, there is still much that can go wrong – transfusion reactions and such like.

Larry was like a lamb and sat still whilst his neck was clipped and prepared for the large needle. Life-saving blood issued down the tube and filled the collection bag, just like it does when we do it, although from the big vein in the neck, rather than a pasty forearm. There was plenty of fussing and plenty of treats for the generous donor.

"That's nearly a whole neck-full," someone called, taking inspiration from the comedian of old, Tony Hancock. "Thank you, Larry – it was better than joining the Young Conservatives," I added, unhelpfully.

The next step was to get the blood into Arianna. A cannula went into the thin vein in her leg and connected to the bag containing Larry's blood. Slowly, the thick fluid, the colour of Merlot, trickled into the little patient and we all watched for signs of reaction. Even a trainee nurse from our practice in Wetherby came to watch and learn, observing for adverse reactions – facial swelling, panting or strange noises. But everything went smoothly and to plan. By midday, Arianna's blood count had increased from nine to thirty-five. We hoped she was fixed; we hoped there'd be no more tears left to cry (which is a line from an Ariana Grande song – sorry!).

CUMC

Last weekend was one of the best. Saturday morning surgery was uneventful and I made it home in time for a lovely spin on my bike. The sunny weather had left all the trails in perfect condition, green buds were appearing on the trees and spring was in the air. The ride was fantastic, but I was late back due to a snapped chain. This messed up the main part of the weekend – a reunion with my old university climbing pals on Saturday night.

Cambridge University Mountaineering Club is one of the oldest and most prestigious climbing clubs in Britain, founded in 1905. I don't think any of its members in the 1990s really appreciated this history. Certainly, very few of us followed in the footsteps of previous climbing greats. But what we lacked in skill we more than made up for in enthusiasm. My time in the club was filled with fun times and great characters. The steep gritstone of Almscliffe Crag, Ilkley and Brimham were excellent training grounds for further forays: winter trips to Ben Nevis or Glen Coe and weekends to the huge and intimidating sea cliffs in Devon and Cornwall. It wasn't long before we had cravings for the bigger peaks of the French and Swiss Alps.

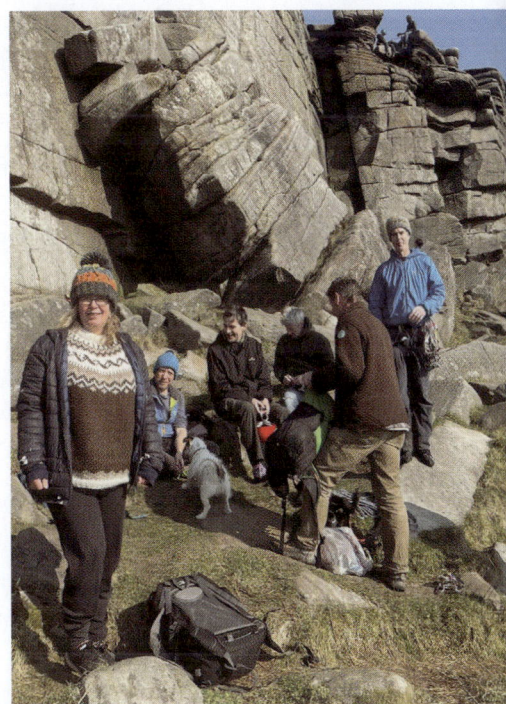

These were happy times for us all, hitching a care-free lift from Cambridge to the Peak District, climbing all day until our hands bled, then drinking until last orders before sleeping in a cave, back at the crag. Of course, for most of us, our studies eventually took priority. I had to concentrate on learning how to become a decent vet and climbing took a back seat. One friend, who was a superb climber and also a mathematics genius, set about a PhD. Reportedly, he cracked the complicated equations in just three weeks but didn't confess, leaving him free to continue his passion for the rocks and crags without the hindrance of university schedules!

So, the chance of a reunion with some of my old friends was hard to resist. Since I had missed the Saturday evening rendezvous because of the chain accident, I arranged to meet them at the crag on Sunday morning. I parked at the bottom and made my way upwards, with Emmy. I'd forgotten how awesome Stanage Edge is, and I felt quite emotional to be back. I was a bit concerned that I might not recognise people whom I had not seen for almost thirty years. I need not have worried. I could spot them from miles away. Tim even had the same helmet, I think, with the same wispy unkempt hair protruding out of the sides.

Apart from one member of the group who had silver hair, everyone looked exactly the same, although I was the only one with the same rock boots. We were an eclectic bunch back then and it was nice to see that the vein of non-conformity continued in some. There was a boat builder, a maths professor and one guy who had a fireworks company. But the best bit was the climbing. I sat on top of the crag, feet dangling groundwards next to the ropes. I'd enjoyed the same view many times before, wishing the sun would hang around so we could stay there longer. As a student, when working in a dusty carpet factory in Wakefield as a holiday job, with the spectre of an unpleasant week's work ahead, I wanted to stay on the sun-drenched rock as long as possible. At least today the prospect of work on Monday morning filled me with as much joy as watching the sunset and reuniting with friends and kindred spirits. It was a great day.

Swan Rescue!

"Are you nearby?" Tracy asked down my phone. I was nearby, on my way back to the practice to cover afternoon surgery. I was pleased to be back to normal veterinary work, after a trip to London the previous day. Channel 5 was celebrating its 25th birthday and I had been fortunate to have been invited along. It was a fantastic evening with lots of highlights. One was standing in the queue to get in next to Tony Robinson, who played Baldrick in *Blackadder*. I resisted the temptation to tell him "I had a cunning plan".

"There is a swan with a bad leg by the river in town. Everyone says you are the expert at catching swans," our practice manager continued. "And Lucy is very keen to help."

"I'll call in to the practice on my way past to pick up some equipment and Lucy," I replied. "I'll be there in five minutes."

It was true, I had previous experience with catching and treating swans. Whether I was an expert was another matter. Famously, one of the first was injured, limping and forlorn. She'd appeared at the nearest house to the lake where she lived, with her mate. The male had knocked on the door with his beak, alerting the humans to the problem. In the dark and under the light of a torch, the dynamic nurse who was helping me jumped into the lake (to where the pair had escaped) and grabbed the swan. Later that evening, we removed a nasty hook which was lodged in the leg.

On another occasion, I'd arrived to find the patient sitting on a small island in the middle of a lake. A neighbour cheerfully volunteered to clamber into a rowing boat to reach the island, capture the swan and return with it, for me to examine. I can't remember exactly how this worked out, but eventually I did examine and treat the bird, which had a nasty carbuncle on its webbed foot.

Today, Lucy and I gathered our equipment and headed to the banks of the river Wharfe. Towels, gloves and even one of those sturdy shopping bags which claim to last a lifetime. They are good for shopping and excellent for enveloping the wings and feet of an ill-tempered swan. We didn't have a spare sock, which was a shame because a large sock is perfect to pop over the head of a swan, to keep it calm and secure the beak.

The river bank, on a warm sunny spring day, was a joyful scene. People sat on benches with ice creams and dogs. Toddlers splashed in frog wellies in the shallow water. There was even a sandy beach! And a lady endlessly and effortlessly fed bread to a swan to persuade it to stay put for the arrival of the emergency team. The swan team; not the swat team. At first, it was hard to ascertain the full extent of the problem and the large, white bird seemed quite happy, gorging itself on bread. The frog-welly-wearing toddler came to help, bending over like toddlers do. "Hello, dog," he said loudly to the swan.

His mum explained that he really, really liked dogs. As the toddler woofed at the swan, it got to its feet and waddled off, like a duck. The left leg was functional but hobbled weakly. I couldn't see any fishing line, nor an obvious hook, but we still needed to capture the patient. Previous experience had taught me that waterfowl have the edge over humans when they get onto the water. There was no time to lose. Lucy unloaded all our equipment and we both stared at the swan, perilously close to the water's edge.

"Lucy," I said. "I have a cunningly plan…"

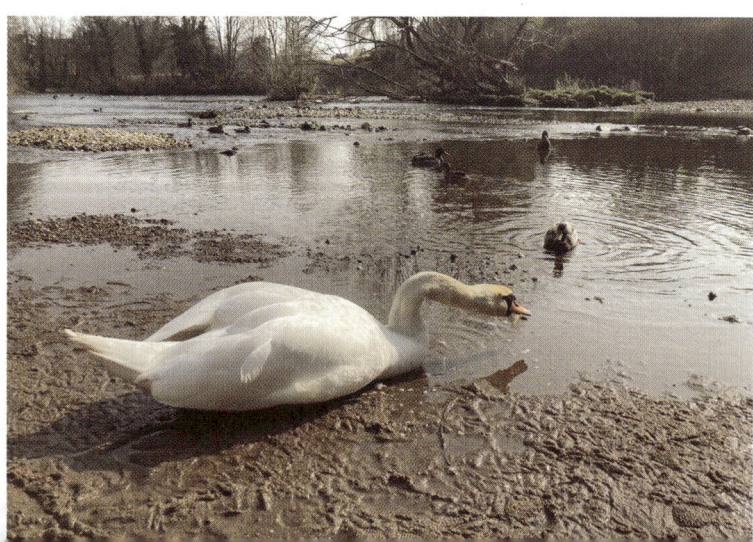

Springtime

It's springtime, which means that *Springtime on the Farm*, a favourite of Channel 5, is back next week. I love this time of year – daffodils, blossom, green shoots of new life, lambs and longer days. The sun has more warmth in its rays and it is a happy time. The programme encapsulates all the hope of spring and it has been fun to be involved since its inception. During the first series, back in 2018, there was live veterinary action in abundance. As we got ready to film an interview in an airy barn made up like a film studio but with straw bales, the telephone of the executive producer started to ring. The walkie-talkie in his other hand was blaring too. A ewe elsewhere on the farm had prolapsed her uterus. This is a life-threatening condition, and I was the only vet on site so it was obvious I needed to attend to the stricken animal.

"But the schedule is tight!" insisted one important telly person, determined to carry on regardless. I objected vigorously, explaining that I could repair the problem within ten or fifteen minutes; and save a life. I'd be back to take my place on the perfectly arranged straw bales within moments. He would have to rearrange his schedule.

Luckily, the energised exec was with me on this one. He agreed that a life *definitely* needed to be saved, ahead of the schedule. I could see the realisation dawning that this was "live" telly and all exciting action would be added interest and excitement for the viewers. And it wouldn't be bad for the viewing figures, either.

"It's chuffing TV gold, Julian," I heard someone bellow, as I grabbed some

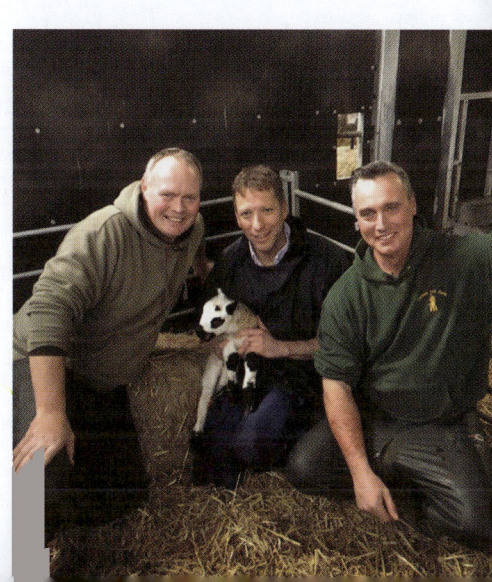

Farmers Rob and Dave, a newborn lamb and me.

kit and ran up to the lambing pens, where Dave the farmer was clutching the ewe's insides to prevent them from spilling on the straw. The next part of the evening was simple for me. I'd done the same procedure hundreds of times before. Ignoring the lights, the cameras and the rest of the action, I was being a vet. That is what I am best at. No retakes, because vets don't get to do retakes. The epidural went smoothly, and I cleaned the prolapsed uterus before replacing it with satisfying ease, finally placing an all-important suture to keep everything in position. I'm not sure how it panned out on TV (I didn't see that bit). I presumed the presenter was offering commentary on the "live stream" that was the sheep's insides and me. I could imagine something like this:

"Julian has just numbed the area with an epidural ... and now he's stopped the ewe from straining he's carefully replacing the uterus ... let's hope it is successful..."

Later that evening, I found myself sitting on straw bales, next to Adam Henson the presenter, with loads of cameras all pointing at me again, some on tripods and one attached to a flying jib, swooping around above and in front of us all.

"How was it up in the lambing pens just now, Julian? It looked very tense?"

"Well, it was a bit stressful, but nothing compared to being interviewed live on television by a famous person off the telly," I wanted to say. Of course, I didn't. Instead, after a deep breath, I explained, as clearly as I could, the ins and outs (or outs and ins, I suppose) of replacing a prolapse in a sheep.

I'm due back to Cannon Hall this week, to help with the next series. There is a call time, a running order and lots of protocols to follow. Maybe there is a tight schedule, too. But you can never adhere to a schedule in the world of veterinary medicine. You never know what is round the next corner.

Stary Smokovec

Stary Smokovec is the closest I have come to visiting Ukraine. At the very Eastern end of a long, cold and (as it was at the time) distinctly Soviet-style train journey from Prague, this was the village from which two friends and I would launch our winter mountaineering forays into the Tatra mountains. This was thirty years ago, and things were very different then. The mountain village was situated in Slovakia, just a few miles from its border with Poland. It was the winter of 1992–93, and for some reason we decided this was the time to explore some new mountains. The Tatra are part of the Carpathian mountain range and offered us something midway between the hills of Scotland and the alpine giants, reaching 2,655 metres at their highest. We left Yorkshire and headed east, with huge rucksacks full of warm clothes, ropes, crampons and ice-axes. Clumpy plastic winter climbing boots gave us the appearance of Power Rangers and an air of invincibility. We decided we were so invincible that we would spend some nights in mountain refuges and the rest in snow holes, carved out of the snowy mountains.

We eventually arrived in Stary, having endured a long night with a Slovakian would-be author, who had written a series of stories, in terrible English, which he hoped to publish. He couldn't believe his luck to be sharing a sleeping compartment with three Brits, even though we were distinctly odd in our strange boots. Into the small and dark hours, he recited one dreadful story after another. He had, apparently, even sent some to the Queen to seek Royal approval.

Our first mountain night was in a refuge on the Polish border. Heated solely by candles – or so it seemed – it was pretty basic, cold and lacking in any sensible conversation between us and the other guests. One of our party could speak German, but in this part of the world, German was not commonly used. Needless to say, we couldn't speak Polish or Czech, nor Slovakian. As soon as we could, we bade our farewells, in the international language of a wave and descended the snowy valley in search of a suitable place to build a snow hole. Luckily, a large hotel quickly came into view, perched on the edge of a very big, frozen and snow-covered lake. It seemed infinitely preferable to a snow hole, so we agreed that, while the three of us were obviously mountain men, we would really rather prefer to stay in a warm hostel. There was more lucky news: there was a room free!

Later, there was more good news, because this particular evening was New Year's Eve and a party was planned. And what a party it was! It coincided with the day that Czechoslovakia separated into two countries – the Czech Republic and Slovakia. Without being able to communicate in a single word, we had the best evening and enjoyed the most fantastic hospitality, sipping from the hip flasks of almost every reveller and singing all the wrong words to their national anthem. The friendliness and inclusion was so palpable and touching. I still remember it with clarity. The three of us were outsiders, aliens in weird, oversized winter climbing boots, with no words to communicate. Yet we were welcomed as friends and with open arms, not as foreign intruders. It's no surprise to see that the communities in this part of the world are doing such an amazing job of helping refugees from their neighbours in Ukraine, fleeing something a whole lot worse than two nights in a snow hole at minus 20.

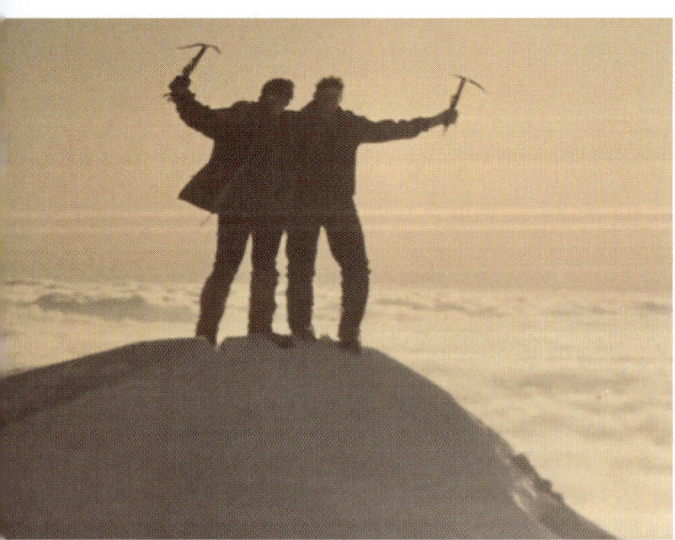

Dave and I, on top of a mountain in the Tatra Mountains in Slovakia, on New Year's Day: their first day as an independent country.

Turn-Out Time

"I've managed to get fifty out already today," said the cheerful farmer, as we chatted at the back of his Land Rover and trailer. He had just lowered the tailgate and waved his arms to encourage the youngsters out and away onto the lush grass. He needn't have bothered with the arm waving, because the black and white bullocks already had a plan. Initially cautious, they quickly developed a taste for adventure with the smell of spring in the air and trotted away in search of their herd mates. There were just four in this load, so I guessed the happy farmer had made many journeys today!

Turn-out is one of the best times of the year for farm animals. The long, dark days of winter have finally passed and cattle can wander freely outside as they are meant to. With less feeding and no bedding to do, the life of the farmer is approaching its best time too. But it is not always without problems. When I worked in Thurso, in the very north of Scotland, turn-out frequently brought its own dangers. After a winter diet which was relatively depleted in vitamin E and selenium – two essential factors in the development of healthy muscles – the sudden burst in activity could lead to a dangerous condition called *white muscle disease*. At its simplest, the effects can be like running a marathon without any training. At its worst, it is a life-threatening problem which can affect the muscles essential for breathing and, worse, the muscle of the heart.

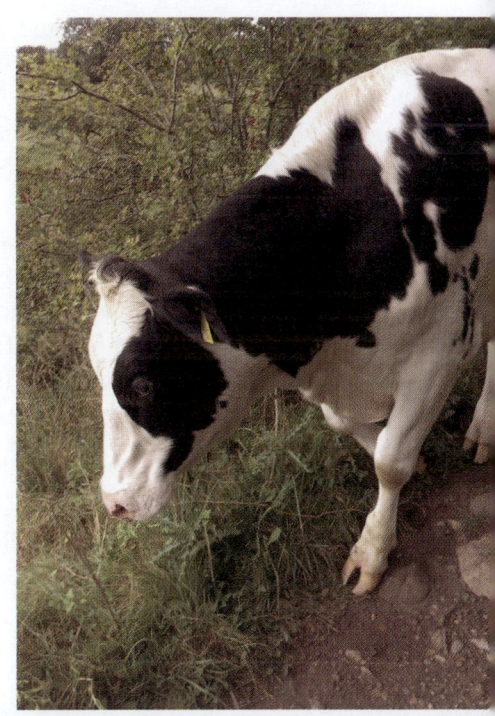

But the turn-out cattle today showed no sign of this as they trotted off with cautious excitement. It reminded me of an occasion, many years ago, when a similar Friesian-cross came a cropper in the very same fields. It had nothing to do with vitamin deficiencies. The ungainly ungulate had tried to negotiate a narrow footbridge. The bridge was designed for people and not cattle, and the animal had slipped, leaving its bulky body on the walkway and its legs dangling down on either side into the ditch below. It couldn't work out how to extricate itself. The vet was called.

That vet on call that evening was recently qualified. This wasn't an eventuality they had covered at vet school and she called for advice. "There's a heifer stuck on a bridge. What can I do?"

As I talked her through the predicament, which had never been described in any veterinary textbook, her beeper went off again – this time a poorly cat.

"Why don't I go and see the heifer on the bridge," I offered, "and you can sort out the cat."

When I arrived, a crowd had gathered. There was a small gang of youths, various dog walkers and two policemen, who had helpfully cordoned off the area with plastic tape, like a crime scene! If I couldn't come up with a plan fairly promptly, it wouldn't be long before there was the white outline of a recently deceased bovine etched on the ground. Luckily, from the far corner of the pasture, a low humming noise could be heard. It was a powerful lifting machine with a big thing on the front, perfect for hoisting cattle. Once it was in place, I organised the crowd to position ropes and straps in such a way as to allow lift-off. Smoke issued from the exhaust pipe and slowly but surely the heifer rose like a phoenix, hovering for several minutes above the river bank and the rest of the cattle.

Once back on the ground, the heifer nonchalantly wandered back to her mates as if nothing had happened. I hoped today's cattle would take care…

Restricted Access

I always enjoy reading Ian McMillan's excellent pieces in the *Yorkshire Post Magazine*, but a recent one struck a particular chord. He described his delight of the discipline enforced by the "550 word limit".

My column, in the *Country Week*, comes in at almost exactly 630 words. Occasionally, it is a stretch to spin out the weekly veterinary anecdotes to fill the space, but more often, the opposite is the case and I need the same discipline to cut out unnecessary words and keep it succinct. Anne is helpful in this regard. She's even better at removing unnecessary punctuation.

Like Ian, who is a true raconteur, I try to follow the general rule that excessive words are annoying and superfluous. A quick look at my clinical veterinary notes over the years will confirm this. The phrase, often added to my clinical notes for a puppy having its first vaccination simply states *fit and well*. This doesn't mean, I hasten to add, that the examination and the check-over was brief – usually quite the opposite in fact. In older dogs, there might be the addition of … *needs dental. Teeth terrible.* Of course, where proper information is required, clinical notes must be more detailed. I'll describe the shape, position and appearance of any abnormality, along with the various differential diagnoses and plans for tests and investigations.

My economy with words started at the outset of my veterinary career. In the olden days, soon after I first started in practice, clinical notes were written by hand on stiff postcards. The date went in the left margin, the notes in the middle and the price on the right-hand side (this had to be calculated quickly, so most medicines were dispensed in multiples of ten to make the maths simpler). There was a general acceptance that words should be kept to a minimum. This was partly to save time but also to save space in the filing cabinet where the card records were kept. More detailed notes led to extra cards being sellotaped together. The general health of any patient could be easily assessed by the thickness of the notes rather than a radiograph. With increasingly detailed notes and an ever-expanding client base, the cabinets bulged to the point where the doors didn't shut.

Back then, a cat, bitten on the tail by a neighbouring tom and suffering from pyrexia and pain, would simply have this jotted on his notes: *CBA, inj BLA*. The position of the CBA was sometimes recorded, but not always.

"CBA" means "Cat Bite Abscess". The next bit referred to the injection of antibiotics. We all knew what and how much to inject into a C with an A to make it better (the BLA bit) as it was a code between vets to save words. Abbreviations were everywhere: ROS (removal of sutures), EAGs (empty anal glands). RFM would often appear in the day book, where there was a similar requirement to save space and to be succinct. It means "retained foetal membranes" and pertains to a recently calved cow with the nasty, smelly and fetid remains of a placenta hanging from her back end.

Nowadays, computers have taken over the role of the postcard, a biro and filing cabinet. They don't have bulging drawers or doors that won't shut. It is simple to make detailed notes and there are usually radiographs and lab results included too. To peruse a patient's clinical record now is sometimes like flicking through an encyclopaedia, with graphs of the dog's weight and reports attached in abundance. The clinical records are undeniably more detailed, and easier to read, but occasionally, when a poorly cat has been in a fight, I'm still tempted to simply write *CBA, inj BLA.* Sometimes there is beauty in brevity.

Boris Has Been Helpful

For once, Boris has been very helpful. Like all of us at this time of year, our haphazard rescued rabbit has a spring in his step. In the sunshine of early May, he has involved himself with some gardening chores, with great enthusiasm. He spends his evenings and nights in his double-decker hutch and his days outside in his capacious pen on the grass, with a tube to run through and various levels to sit on to keep things interesting. However, if we are all at home and the gate can be kept securely locked, he is allowed out to run around the garden, investigate flavoursome bushes (his favourite is a hebe) and relax in the sun.

He's an interesting character, verging on the completely dozy. We acquired him as a rescue a few years ago, after someone found him and handed him into the practice. We have no idea how old he is, but our best guess is about seven, so quite old. He and our other rabbit Luna truly loved one another, but sadly we lost Luna last year, leaving Boris by himself. Luckily, he is easily pleased and happy in his own company.

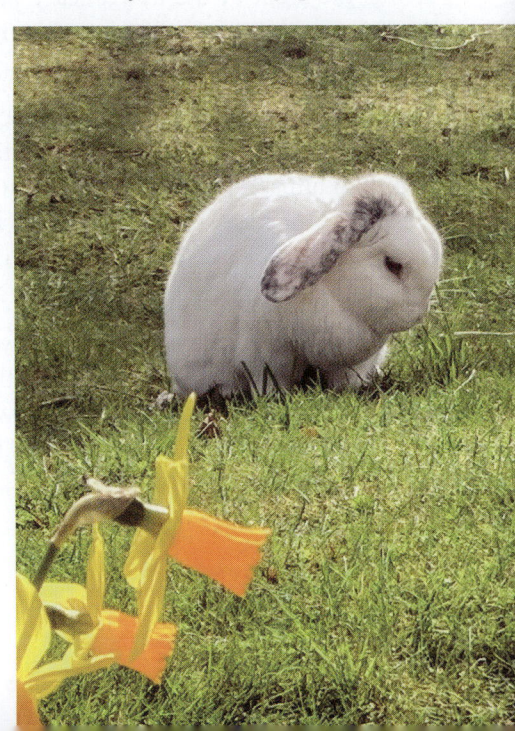

He was most helpful today with the process of removing an overgrown herbaceous plant, which left a large hole in the shrubbery. When he thought no human was looking, the floppy lop took himself to the middle of the patch of soil, where he would dig furiously – like only rabbits and terriers do – before stopping and throwing himself flat on his side, as if he'd suddenly had a heart attack. He would lie motionless for a few moments, then would wriggle himself into an upright position before repeating the same trick on his other side. He seemed to be enjoying himself. What Boris didn't know was that we were all watching from the kitchen, laughing our heads off! I often wonder what goes on in the heads of our pets.

Fortunately, he was not interested in the reseeded patches of lawn, apart from performing some excavations of his own around the edges, but Boris became very animated when the scabious flowers were planted. He liked the taste of the leaves as well as the flowers. Anne quickly erected a rabbit-proof fence to keep him at whiskers' length. The best bit of his day though, was a brief foray into the vegetable patch. This is usually a part of our garden where Boris is not allowed to go, so he became excited the moment he hopped through the gate. Everyone knows that a rabbit in a vegetable patch can lead to disaster. Anyone who grew up with *Peter Rabbit* and the *Flopsy Bunnies* is well aware of the peril. But Boris was not distracted by lettuces or radishes (which had not yet been planted). It was the sight of the newly leafy parsley in the far corner that made his rabbit eyes light up and he made a beeline for the herb. Peter Rabbit would have been proud!

Later, I sat with him and helped pluck and brush away some of his winter coat. He is getting quite stiff these days and struggles to groom himself properly, so we need to keep a close eye on him. He looked much smarter by the time I had finished and there was a satisfyingly large pile of white fluff on the grass: a perfect material for lining birds' nests!

We'd all had a nice day, enjoying the warmth of springtime. On the newly mowed lawn, as the sun was dipping low, Boris continued to hurtle about with bursts of energy which defied his old age. He leapt up in the air with nifty side flips like a young lamb. He liked his tidy new coat.

Gerald, Thomas and Christopher

The Town Crier was shouting his head off and ringing his bell loudly. "Oh, yay. Oh yay!" he bellowed as the gong clanged.

This was the signal for Mr Mayor and me to emerge from the little church to join the assembled group of cat fans. I was slightly anxious because I had never unveiled a statue before. In the brief chat with the mayor beforehand, it transpired that he hadn't either. So, we were both novices. I looked around for the monument, which was smaller than I expected and hidden under a bag. For some reason, I was expecting something like the lions in Trafalgar Square. I composed myself, said a few words and then removed the bag with a flourish to reveal Gerald to the world.

Gerald was a cat, and the Yorkshire-stone sculpture had been handcrafted in his image to commemorate his life. The charismatic Bengal had spent much of his time patrolling the grounds of York Minster and the nearby Holy Trinity Church, where he is now immortalised.

The affection with which the gathered crowd spoke about Gerald after the unveiling was remarkable. Gerald went out of his way to meet, greet and befriend visitors to York, and he had a large fan base of visitors and local residents alike. It reminded me again just how much impact animals can have on our lives. All cat owners will concur that the feline/human bond is a unique one.

Gerald's story and his legacy reminded me of another cat whose presence carried significance for many. Thomas Gray was a sleek black and white tomcat who lived at Pembroke – my college at Cambridge, where I went to vet school. Named after the English poet, who was a professor at Pembroke, the cat prowled around the tranquil grounds of the historic college in the same way, I imagine, as Gerald had done in York. He remained aloof and totally oblivious to the amount of time any of us spent in either the library or the college bar. He was friends with many of the undergraduates,

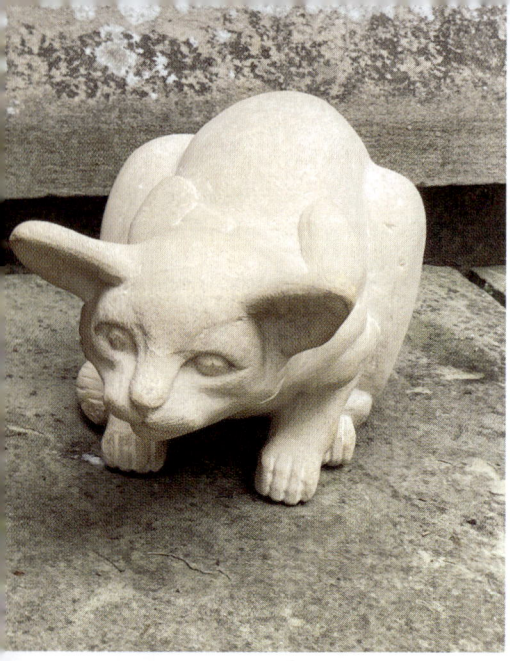

but not especially close to anyone. I'm sure he had seen it all before.

The most regarded poem written by the human Thomas Gray was called *Elegy Written in a Country Churchyard*, which seemed apt as I admired Gerald's sculpture in the grounds of Holy Trinity Church, especially as the evocative poem alludes to the desire of humans (but not necessarily cats) to be remembered after their death.

The ceremony concluded and I said my goodbyes to the mayor, Gerald and all the people connected to Holy Trinity Church. It was an interesting church, with ancient box pews that apparently are now very rare, and I would have liked to explore more but I needed to get back to proper veterinary work, which was very likely to involve actual, live cats.

Later that evening, I decided to delve a little further. I discovered that the demise of the box pew was all because of Sir Christopher Wren, who was the pre-eminent church designer of the late 1600s (think St Paul's Cathedral). He didn't like them and so they fell out of fashion. As I read on, it occurred to me that this was an amazing coincidence, because Sir Christopher Wren had also designed the chapel of Pembroke College, Cambridge, where Thomas Gray (the cat *and* the poet) and I had spent many happy years. I could never have imagined that the unlikely and unusual occasion of unveiling a cat statue could have yielded so many inter-connected stories.

Sponge Bob; Square Stomach

"Sponge Bob is back," Sarah, our smiley receptionist called. "He's coming in about twenty minutes. Is that OK?" Her grin defied the seriousness of Sponge Bob's situation, although it was impossible not to see the funny side of this vizsla's predicament.

Sponge Bob wasn't his real name, rather the nickname we'd given to him after the previous accidental swallowing. For no obvious reason, on that occasion, the youngster had eaten a whole sponge. One of those green ones, the size of a bar of soap, with a scouring surface on one side. These things don't show up easily on an X-ray, so the endoscope was the tool of choice to establish if the sponge was actually inside the patient. It's generally quite important to ascertain with certainty that the foreign body has definitely been swallowed. I once spent several afternoons radiographing a Border collie whose gummy owner had lost his false teeth. The elderly gentleman was adamant that Floss has swallowed them, but repeated radiographs failed to confirm this. There were various loops of bowel which seemed to be grinning at us on the X-ray film, but none that were conclusive enough to justify surgery. Eventually, the teeth turned up. They had fallen down the back of the bedside table, so it was a good job we didn't operate on Floss.

With the endoscope, we quickly found the sponge, which was hiding under a thick layer of gastric bubbles (perhaps the sponge had recently been used to clear up washing-up liquid?). After many minutes of attempting to get a good enough hold to remove the scouring pad with the endoscope

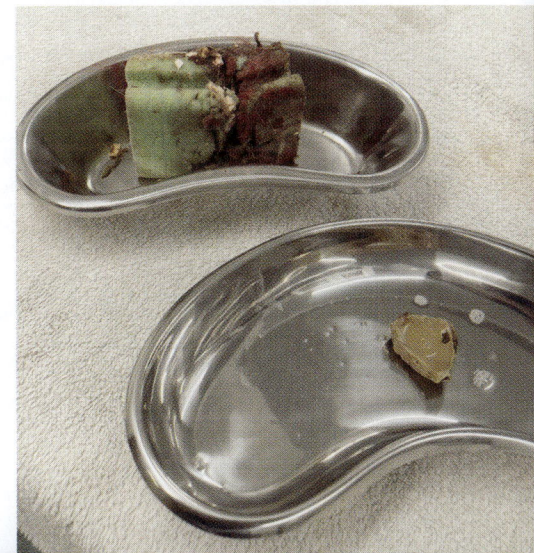

grabbers, it became apparent that the sponge was only coming out in small pieces. It was too big and too wedged to reverse out whole. Surgical intervention was required. Sponge Bob was wheeled into theatre.

He made a complete and uneventful recovery after that first sponge-removal surgery, but we were very surprised that he was on his way back just a few weeks later suffering from exactly the same predicament. He looked every bit as happy and healthy as usual. His tail wagged with delight – he seemed to love his visits to the vet's. He had a nonchalant yet triumphant air.

"And he's *definitely* eaten it?" I asked his owner, always harking back to the curious incident of the false teeth *not* in the dog. I wanted to make sure this was no wild goose chase.

"Definitely. He grabbed it in his mouth. I tried to get it from him but when he saw me, he just swallowed it down in one! I'm certain it's inside him," came the confirmation. "It's exactly the same as the one he swallowed last time. They come in packets of three."

There was no need for X-rays and I knew endoscopy would not help. I also knew that sponges like this inside a vizsla could only be removed surgically – the rough surface clings on to the wall of the stomach or intestine like Velcro, and the sponge can swell dangerously – so it was a case of history repeating itself. Again, everything went to plan and the process was much simpler without first trying to hoist it out with the 'scope.

He came back in today, for his stitches to be removed. The wound had healed perfectly and the young vizsla was back to full health.

"This wound looks great!" I said, removing each suture in turn, "Have you found another way of cleaning the dishes? Maybe a brush? Or a dishwasher?"

"Yes. And we've thrown out the other sponge. It won't be happening again!"

Stories from Scotland (1)

Another veterinary practice is back in the spotlight at the moment. McGregor and Partners, the UK's most northerly practice in Thurso, is the venue for Channel 5's *The Highland Vet*. Whether it is a pure coincidence that this was the practice in which I cut my teeth as a young vet or not, I'm still not sure. From my time there, I know there is a rich vein of characters and stories and the backdrop is just as beautiful as anything Yorkshire has to offer. But making a TV series so far north must have been a huge challenge. Whilst the summer months enjoy long days with huge skies and far-reaching views over distant hills and rugged coastlines, the hibernal gloom makes winter a grim time of year up in Caithness. Darkness and rain are the enemies of television producers and directors. And there is an abundance of both from October to March.

Another challenge to making reality documentaries is the audio. Strong winds play havoc with sound quality and heavy accents can leave viewers confused or perplexed. I remember when I worked in Caithness I sometimes needed a translator. It was a wild, rugged place and the work was equally tough. It was not uncommon to spend a whole day castrating cattle who had never seen a vet before and hardly knew what a human being was. And as for calving and lambing time! A steady stream of farmers would appear at the end of the afternoon, with trailers full of sheep to lamb. There was a slick production line for caesarean sections – the skilful vets could complete a caesar in less than ten minutes.

It was a perfect place for a young vet to learn the ropes. I performed my first, solo cow caesarean in a dark cow byre in the small hours. It went to plan and my confidence grew by the day. Of course, there were setbacks too. One morning, a farmer appeared with two ewes in the back of his trailer, both with bulging prolapses. During coffee time (a rare event, but I recall several vets and receptionists were all in the same place at the same time) I volunteered to go into the car park to sort them out. "It should be simple," I thought.

It would have been simple, had the two sheep not jumped over the flimsy tailgate and completed a lap of the car park before running off up the small road where the practice resided. If the pair had turned left, they would have quickly arrived in the town square of Thurso, where my embarrassment would have been complete. Luckily, they turned right and headed past some houses and on to a long and quiet lane, fenced on both sides. The taciturn farmer and I followed, hotly and with increasing levels of exasperation. He couldn't get past the ewes to head them off. Eventually, and I'm not sure how, the sheep ended up in a ditch, where I managed to jump on top and restrain them both using all arms and legs. The red-faced farmer marched back to get his vehicle. As he disappeared into the distance, I was sure I could see steam still coming from his ears.

The repair of the prolapses was simple after that but completed in the absence of any conversation with the furious farmer. I tried to remain calm and friendly and waved him off, thanking my lucky stars that nothing worse had happened. I returned to the staff room several hours later, where coffees had long been finished.

"How did the prolapses go?" asked one of the senior vets, mindful that I'd been absent all morning. "Don't worry. They sometimes do take ages. You'll get quicker the more you do"

I nodded, thanked him and kept quiet.

Stories from Scotland (2)

Memories from the beginning of my veterinary career in Scotland have kept coming. My three-month sojourn saw my confidence soaring, but every week there was a minor catastrophe to bring me back to earth. And each one was a lesson learnt.

In my third week, I had to perform a post-mortem examination on a suddenly dead stirk. I'm sure there was a term in local dialect for a stirk, but I can't remember what it was. (Cows, for example, were often called something which sounded like "Coo-wa-gie", while any female human was respectfully called a "wifey"). Anyhow, I knew from vet school that it was essential to undertake an anthrax test on any bovine which had died suddenly and inexplicably. A small smear of blood was removed from an ear and examined, cow-side, with special stain and a microscope. If the carcass was free of Bacillus anthracis then it was safe to perform a post-mortem. Cutting open an anthrax-ridden carcass risked exposing the farm and the whole area to the deadly spores.

I grabbed the practice microscope and headed out equipped with saws, knives and big rubber gloves.

"Hang on," shouted the cheerful senior vet, "I need the microscope for an itchy dog. I shouldn't worry about doing an anthrax test. They always come back negative." Deferring to his experience, I pressed on and once I'd got to the farm, duly set about the autopsy on the recently deceased creature, which was lying next to the muck heap. It was a dangerous job. Between cuts I had to waft my arms to defend myself from clouds of malevolent midges, which sensed my young, tasty English flesh.

Inside was a bloody mess. The spleen was huge; blood was everywhere and even frothed and bubbled from the poor animal's mouth. Its demise had been so swift there was no trace of *rigor mortis* – a sure sign of septicaemia. I collected samples into a plastic bag and loaded everything into the little van I'd been given to use for my locum job. I felt a bit like Postman Pat, though with a more unusual parcel.

Finally, I cast an eye over the rest of the group, taking the temperatures of a few animals. They were all sky high. I agreed to perform some tests and report back post-haste.

On my way back to the practice, I pulled into a small car park by a beautiful beach to consider the clues. "If that was a spleen, it was enormous. Why was there no *rigor mortis*? The blood from the mouth; the extremely high temperatures in the others. I flicked through my textbook and looked in the infectious disease section under "A".

As I scanned through the list of clinical signs, I started to fear I had made the worst veterinary mistake ever. I looked in the rear-view mirror and scratched my now-blistering face. The final clinical sign on the page was one seen in humans: acute skin lesions. Followed by immediate death.

By now I felt certain it was not just my veterinary career that was about to be cut short prematurely. I went for a final walk on the long and deserted beach. I sat on a rock and looked out to sea. Not far away was Gruinard Island, the site of testing for biological warfare where anthrax was tested in the Second World War. I feared the worst. Eventually, I plucked up courage and delivered the bag of entrails to the desk of the local lab.

"I've just been to see a dead stirk. Its organs are in this bag. I think I've just made a terrible mistake."

Luckily, I hadn't. The calves had peracute pneumonia. And my blistered face? Nothing more than the effects of *Culicoides impunctatus*: the Scottish midge!

Oystercatcher

We've had an oystercatcher at the practice in Thirsk this week. Fortunately, the beautiful black and white bird was not physically injured, so there was no need for any veterinary intervention. He was strutting about outside, initially confidently and cockily but eventually confused. Did he need attention, I wondered?

Narcissus, as we quickly named the bird, was looking for a mate. In fact, he was looking at his mate. His mate was seemingly *inside* the practice and was making exactly the same moves that he was making, on the other side of the gleaming glass front door. Nobody had the heart to tell Narcissus the truth – he was lusting after his own reflection – so he hung around, unrequited, for almost a week. His favourite time to impress his own reflection was in the evening. It was quiet and the light was just right.

This was not the first time I'd witnessed a story of a bird outside a door. Some years ago, I'd seen a male and female swan who had appeared late one evening outside the house nearest to the lake where they lived. The larger bird, the male, had (apparently) knocked on the door with his beak, alerting the humans inside to a problem. The problem was Mrs Swan, who was hobbling with a painful leg. The story sounds implausible, but the young daughter in the house had captured the door-knocking birds on her phone, as all good teenagers do these days. The evidence was irrefutable. After politely knocking, both birds moved back a few webbed footsteps and waited for the humans to answer. The female obligingly lifted her injured leg at exactly the correct moment to indicate that her leg was injured. Having raised the alarm, the pair of love birds swiftly retired to the inky lake. As darkness fell, the humans called the surgery and I overheard the odd telephone conversation with the receptionist.

"There's a pair of swans on your doorstep? And they've knocked on the door? And one is injured? And now they've returned to the lake? In the darkness?" I grabbed the equipment I thought I might need and persuaded the most willing and capable nurse on hand – Sarah – to join me on the quest. Arriving at the lake in pitch darkness, fifteen minutes later, the task of finding an injured swan seemed impossible. The homeowners next to the lake recounted the story but shrugged their shoulders when questioned about the birds' whereabouts. Was this a wild goose chase? Moments later, we realised possibly not. The swans were just about visible, bobbing around in the water by its edge. Without any thought of personal safety, Sarah leapt into the dark water like a salmon and grabbed the nearest bird. Luckily, this was the injured female. Even in the dark, with the help of a head torch, we could see that there was a fishing hook deeply embedded in her leg. I quickly judged that it would need removal under general anaesthetic, so there was an uncomfortable trip back to the operating theatre. The hook came out quite easily, although avoiding the important blood vessels and tendons needed care.

The following morning, early before normal work resumed, we returned Mrs Swan to the lake. On a misty morning, with a weak winter sun just rising, the lake had an Arthurian air. There was an emotional reunion as the husband calmly glided over to meet us. The two love birds embraced by intertwining their necks before swimming away.

"Where have you been? And how's your leg?" I imagined the conversation went. It left me pondering the origins of the phrase *Bird Brain*.

Benzene Ring

There were just three more people left to see at the end of a manic Monday. To begin with, it had looked as if it was shaping up to be a quiet day, with two ops cancelled at the last minute due to illness and vehicular breakdown. This unusual scenario was altered abruptly by the arrival, in close succession, of a cat hit by a car and a Staffie with a bloody nasal discharge. X-rays, pins and screws, drips, endoscopy, biopsies and more X-rays ensued. As the afternoon drew to a close, a new puppy for vaccines, a re-bandage for a pesky tail injury and a health check for a newly registered client was all that stood in the way of home time.

"Sherlock, please," I called, looking out of my consulting room at the likely candidates waiting patiently. Instinctively, I was drawn to the cute and chunky puppy, but that was not Sherlock. The pup's owners shook their heads and looked in the direction of the real Sherlock. So did I, and that was when I gasped. The gasp was immediately followed by a huge grin. I recognised the Border collie's owner immediately, even though I had not seen her for over three decades. There, right in front of me, was my chemistry teacher from approximately thirty-two years ago. We'd become good friends back then, sharing a passion for both chemistry and outdoor pursuits. When I was seventeen, benzene rings and climbing mountains were my main fascinations and Sherlock's owner had shared similar interests.

Sherlock was her latest in a long line of Border collies. The first one I knew was an amazing dog, called Laska. Her energy was infectious, and she accompanied us all on mountaineering and climbing trips across the Dales and beyond. Only recently, I discovered the origin of this collie's name. It was taken from a canine character in Tolstoy's classic novel *Anna Karenina*. It turns out, having read the book and known the dog, that the Laska from Leeds shared many characteristics with Tolstoy's Laska. Enthusiastic, experienced and dedicated, Tolstoy's version quickly becomes impatient and excited as her master, a country gentleman, gets organised for a day's shooting. Fantastically, Tolstoy describes how Laska senses her master's misfortune and dismay at missing his birds. She doesn't want to show any lack of faith in her master's ability, so she pretends to search for the birds, just to please him. It's a wonderful moment in the epic story.

We quickly covered the Tolstoy connection, before moving onto chemistry, old times and old friends. The Sponsored Three Peaks of Great Britain expedition held fond and terrible memories for both of us; starting our ascent of Ben Nevis with little or no sleep was a low point (only Laska seemed delighted to be outside that morning, so very, very early). Reaching the summit before midday, having raised hundreds of pounds – which was a lot back then – was the high point, quite literally.

"I remember you once running down the corridor, waving a piece of paper above your head, shouting 'I've worked it out! I've got the answer,'" she recounted.

"I don't remember that. What was the answer?" I asked. Apparently, it was something to do with a chemical structure of a derivative of benzoic acid.

Again, times had changed. Once, the structure of a derivative of benzoic acid had been all-important for us both. Now, more importantly, I needed to find out if there was anything wrong with Sherlock, another dog named after a literary character. It was time to look for clues…

Dog Treats

We have some healthy dog treats in the practice now. They were acquired with the aim of persuading dogs that it's a lovely idea to come to the vet's. With the added benefit of improving dental health, the combination seemed ideal. A special treat, which isn't a treat at all, but morsels of dentally perfect dog food. Genius! But unfortunately, this tactic of dental care by stealth did not meet with the approval of most of the canines. The canine patients, I mean. Not the canine teeth.

I've never been a fan of bribery and I'm not totally convinced about offering snacks to all our patients. Vets spend much of their time talking about the importance of weight management and the implications of carrying extra pounds. I've never been to the doctors and come out with a lolly or a doughnut. That said, it's an undeniably different experience visiting a vet – not least where we put our thermometers – so I suppose a spoonful of sugar and all that.

One patient came in this week with her own food for the day. It was to be offered after she had recovered from her anaesthetic. The gourmet package looked tasty and was called "Nature's Canine Kitchen Garden Pantry", or something similar. It looked as delicious as it seemed wholesome. I was almost tempted to grab a forkful.

"That packet costs four pounds," commented one of the nurses. My jaw dropped. It was more expensive than my own lunch would be, whenever that time arrived. Later in the morning, I saw a young poodle-cross called Mitzi. A poor appetite and intermittent vomiting seemed to be the main problems, although Mitzi otherwise looked a picture of health. An interesting conversation followed, again focused on food.

"We've tried all sorts of food, but she just doesn't seem to like any of them," the worried owner explained, shaking her head as she spoke. "We've tried them all."

The husband quickly added, "And the new one we've got is so hard, I have to hit it with a hammer." I raised my eyebrows. No food I had ever come across – for dogs, humans or any other creature – needed to be bashed like this. Maybe this was the reason Mitzi was not an enthusiastic eater?

It was all a far cry from days gone by. My grandparents kept dogs and ran a small boarding kennels. I have crystal-clear memories of dogs' dinners back in the day. A huge, dented metal bowl would appear from the "coal house". It was no longer a coal house by then, but was filled with dog leads, wellies, dog food, gardening tools and large, metal bowls for mixing food. My gran would shovel handfuls of biscuit-like, pebble-sized nuggets (called "mixer") into the bowl and stir it up with several enormous tins of pasty dog food. It had a consistency (and probably a similar composition) somewhere between spam and meat paste. The aroma was more difficult to describe. After about five minutes of mixing, the delicious concoction was ready and was shared out into smaller bowls for all the hungry dogs. It disappeared in seconds, leaving the bowls spotless. I couldn't help but wonder what Mitzi would have made of that. It certainly didn't need to be hit with a hammer and it *definitely* didn't cost four pounds a portion!

I examined Mitzi and failed to identify any obvious problems, before explaining a possible course of action. We agreed to carry out some X-rays (to check for something like a pebble stuck in the stomach) and some blood tests (to rule out Addison's disease and other bad things) and we booked Mitzi in for the next day.

As they headed back to their car, I noticed Mitzi's owners had picked up a packet of "tasty-but-healthy-dog-dental-treats" to add to Mitzi's smorgasbord. I hoped it would work.

Getting Old?

We enjoyed a lovely weekend of celebrating recently. The combination of sunny weather, the wedding of a friend and colleague and a significant birthday saw a large surge in my cake consumption, not to mention wine. Luckily, it was for only one (long) weekend. One cannot survive exclusively on wine and cake for very long. As one of the first birthday cards said: *The years have been extremely kind to you. It's the weekends that have done the damage.*

We were nearly late for the wedding – a bassett with a strip of fabric tangled in its bowel and a Dalmatian with a pine cone in his, followed by a collie in need of a stitch-up took us right up to the last possible minute. The final sutures were placed and followed by the most rapid of quick changes, like Superman and Wonder Woman, although with very different outfits. The taxi driver, who was tapping his fingers on the steering wheel whilst waiting outside our house, was visibly impressed.

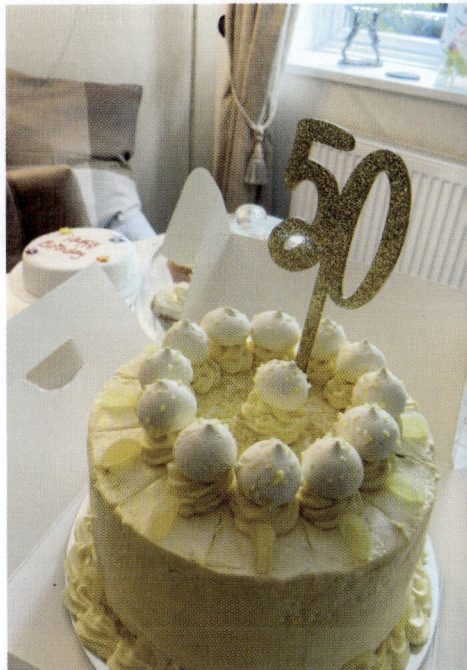

I don't feel fifty, so it was confusing when almost all the cards appeared to have that number written on the front. "I wonder who all those cards are for" was my first and recurring thought when I caught sight of them. At least I could catch sight of them. Depleted eyesight is one of the early signs of "getting on" and I'm fighting the need to get some of those glasses that you can buy from the supermarket rather than an optician. I know they are good, if not essential and

I also know it's only a matter of time. Close-up surgery can be frustrating but luckily the table or the patient can usually be moved further away. The tiny print on the menus of dimly lit restaurants present the biggest problem. I can sympathise with a friend who was once perusing the list of pizzas on offer at a local Italian when we went out for dinner.

"I think I'd like this one at the bottom, please," he pronounced to the waiter. On closer inspection, the writing at the bottom started by saying: "Additional toppings." It was followed by a long list of every single possible pizza accoutrement, which clearly looked a delicious combination when viewed completely out of focus.

Compared to some, my eyes are faring OK, although fastening the safety pin on the back of the badge which proudly stated "50 today" proved sufficiently challenging that I had to pull a funny face to focus. I suppose I could have attached the badge a bit lower down.

I'm pretty fit and I'm pleased to say I can almost keep up with my teenage kids at some sports. Last week, when Jack and I raced around the trails near Thirsk on our mountain bikes, had I not stopped to pick up a stray banana skin I might even have come home first. It's harder to beat Archie, although left-handed table tennis appears to be his Achilles heel. I once remember seeing a parent failing to keep up with his seven-year-old daughter during a fun run and it focused my mind, not least to try and set a good example.

If you ask Anne, she'll say that my age-related failure is primarily affecting my ears. I do not agree. I think she should speak a little louder and not at times when other loud things are happening. Having said that, when asked just now before a short dog walk if I could pass her a poo bag, I must have looked confused.

"Why do you want a *shoe bag*?" I replied. Her eyes rolled upwards. "A POO bag!" she bellowed this time, before collapsing in a heap of laughter.

Yew Turn

I took a deep breath. It was certainly the largest thing I'd ever tried to remove. It had grown slowly. Maybe it should have been cut out earlier, when it was smaller. It would have been a simpler task. I pondered which of the laid-out instruments to use first. Instinctively, I reached for the saw, before thinking better of it.

"If I can just reduce its bulk first," I thought and put down the saw. The loppers would surely be a better choice. "If I can get those lower branches off it's less likely to hit me on the head when I eventually use the axe."

As the branches tumbled around me, I felt sad because I don't like cutting down trees. But over the last eighteen years, the once-small bush had totally outgrown its place and it needed to go. Even worse, its needle-like leaves contained an important and powerful chemical and it seemed wasteful not to make the most of its medicinal properties. I'm sure I remember in the past that people used to collect the fallen branches of Yew trees and send them to pharmaceutical companies; the ultimate in recycling. Or is it upcycling? But I'd searched everywhere online and this doesn't seem to be a thing anymore. It's not economical. Yew is full of chemicals called taxines. Most are dangerous and cause rapid death as a result of toxicity to the heart. All vets who work with cattle have examined mouths and rumens during a post-mortem for signs of the spikey evergreen. It's a classic cause of unexpected death if cattle or sheep browse the wrong greenery. Some of these chemicals, however, can be converted into anti-cancer medication, notably the drug tamoxifen. Apparently, it takes six one-hundred-year-old yew trees to treat one cancer patient, which explains why they don't collect it from yew trees anymore.

But yew is not the only plant filled with powerful drugs. Periwinkles provide great ground cover and look pretty with lovely little lilac flowers (until they take over your flower beds and strangle everything else). They also make cool chemicals called vinca-alkaloids, from which the staple chemotherapy drugs vincristine and vinblastine derive. I've injected countless vials into dogs suffering from lymphoma over the years. Foxgloves are jam-packed with digitalis, a great drug for treating a heart condition called atrial fibrillation. The list of plant-derived medicines is almost endless; aspirin from the bark of willow trees – discovered as far back as the eighteenth century; morphine from a brown resin in poppy plants; atropine – the mouth-drying and pupil-dilating drug – from deadly nightshade, otherwise known as *belladonna* because the effects of making the pupils large was thought (at least by Cleopatra) to make them more alluring.

Step sideways from the plant kingdom to the wonderful world of fungi and there is another bewilderingly huge list of medicines. Penicillin – the first antibiotic; cyclosporin – the first immunosuppressant to make transplant surgery a possibility; and statins, now lowering cholesterol and apparently extending the lives of cheese-lovers indefinitely.

The pile of removed branches was getting bigger and the tree correspondingly smaller. Although that corner of the garden was looking bare, it was a job nearly well done. I piled up the bigger branches and shoved the clippings into the green recycling bin until it was full, then promptly jumped in. This was a habit I had picked up from a former work colleague who, despite his seniority, would jump into the rubbish bin each week using a small set of steps, to squash down the rubbish. It saved space and a few quid.

One jam-packed wheelie bin and a large pile of logs. I reckoned that would treat approximately one tenth of a cancer patient, which I felt sure was better than nothing. It seemed a shame to turn it into compost.

Birthday Ziggy

Consulting non-stop from two o'clock until six-thirty on an afternoon seems to be a regular occurrence at the moment. A combination of our veterinary practices being popular and a national shortage of veterinary manpower means that most days are very busy, often without the chance to stop for a coffee, or even a wee. This is a good thing though (not the lack of toilet breaks), because it's better to be busy. Having said that, I'm not sure how next Monday is going to work out, with an ops list extending off the page and already including three complicated surgeries. We'll cross that bridge when we come to it…

Today followed the same pattern of a full list with extras squeezed in. The final appointment of the afternoon threatened to eat into the time that we set aside for cleaning, but instead of the usual *vomiting and diarrhoea* or *scratching* written beside the animal's name, it said

Ziggy, birthday. Bringing prosecco and cake.

It seemed Ziggy wasn't even poorly!

It was his birthday – of course! Unfortunately, we hadn't had a chance to arrange any wine glasses, let alone order the party poppers. As the cork popped, the fizzy beverage was carefully poured into mugs to raise the toast. After a busy day it seemed an excellent compensation for the lack of coffee.

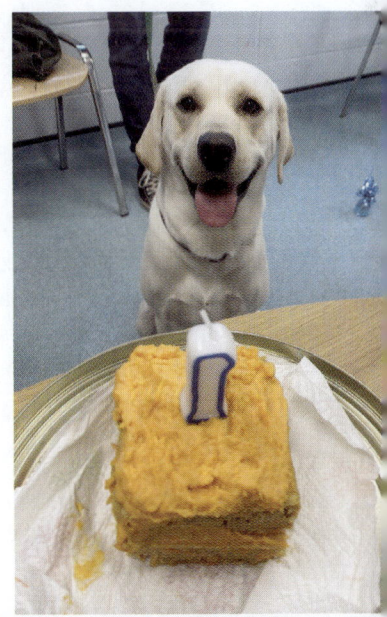

There was a "happy first birthday" helium-filled balloon and a special dog cake. A cake for dogs, rather than a cake in the shape of a dog. Obviously. Ziggy's owner had put a candle on top, although it became evident that this was not a great idea for a dog, as he didn't understand how to blow it out, and just wanted to get on with the eating. Various photos were taken with the assembled guests and toasts were raised. Ziggy wagged his tail and tucked into his special cake, with enthusiasm.

"It's exactly a year since you delivered him, Julian," explained Ziggy's owner, holding her mug of prosecco in the air. I have to admit, I hadn't remembered exactly the details, but fortunately she jogged my memory.

"His mum was struggling to give birth. She'd had four or five pups during the day – Charlie, Humphrey, Freddie and Booboo – but Ziggy was stuck. Mum was exhausted and her contractions had fizzled out. Anne had been dealing with it, but she had to go for her Covid jab and you were drafted in at the last minute to do an emergency caesarean. If it wasn't for you he wouldn't be here. He wouldn't be celebrating his first birthday!"

Now I remembered! I'd rushed back from Sandbeck as evening surgery was coming to a close to help out. It was back in the first few months of our Thirsk practice being open. A time when everything was a blur. Like a supercharged sports car, the practice had gone from nought to sixty in about as many days. Every day was hectic as new clients and old faces flooded in. At the time, I felt that we were all riding the wave with composure, but evidently some of it disappeared from my memory in the whirl. A lot has changed in a year. Thirsk Veterinary Centre feels like a long-established practice, with fabulous clients and pets and ops lists replete with all manner of investigations and treatments. We have a cohort of lovely staff who feel like family and have helped to train two veterinary nurses. We've saved lives and brought new life into the world. One of whom was standing right in front of me, polishing off the final morsels of dog cake until there was just an inedible candle left. Happy Birthday Ziggy. It's been a good first year!

Sheep on Hay Bales

Previously, I've made vague reference to the task of choosing topics for this column and, once chosen, the joy of creating a succinct summary of the subject. This week's subject matter came out of the blue, after a literary festival in Hexham.

"Can I show you some pictures from my album?" said an energetic lady (who I will call Fiona, although that wasn't her actual name) as she presented me with two books to sign. "I think you might be interested."

"I've been collecting photos which I've taken during winter bike rides around the Northern Dales," she explained. "They are all of sheep on hay bales." Sure enough, there was a large collection of photos of sheep standing on and around hay bales and at ring feeders. The best ones, or at least the ones about which Fiona became most excited, were the ones with sheep standing on top of a central bale.

As I flicked through the niche portfolio, Fiona continued to explain her aims and motives and the challenges associated with photographing sheep on bales of hay:

"My target for next winter is to add more to the collection," she enthused. "January and February are the best months, and 2018 and 2019 were my best cycling winters for sheep on hay bale photography. Since then the album's growth has slowed, because I have either been too cold to remove all of my gloves or its been too wet to take my phone out of its waterproof bag – sheep on hay bale photography is a savage, brutal hobby, you know."

I nodded in agreement. I could only imagine, although I do have some experience of photographing sheep (mainly for use in this column), so I could sympathise.

Fiona continued to outline more of the challenges involved in trying to capture the perfect ovine scene:

"Sometimes the sheep get scared or frightened by my shrieks of delight (which are meant to be encouraging, not frightening, but they don't know that), and jump off the hay bale. On other occasions, there simply haven't been the photographic opportunities, even when a hay bale has been ripe for climbing. Maybe the sheep on those occasions were lazy?"

We chatted more, before I added my signature to the books. I apologised for the lack of photographs of sheep on bales in each book, but I jotted my email address on the inside cover of one and promised to peruse her pictures in more detail if she sent them by email. Later, a series of photos duly appeared, along with some further explanation, which went like this:

Apart from sheep on hay bales, I take no photographs, so my knowledge of how photo sharing works is negligible. I hope I have attached three of my favourites:

The only one I took last winter (the one with the house in the background) is my absolute favourite. Initially, when we saw this sheep, I thought I was hallucinating or my packed lunch had been drugged, because it was too good to be true.

Another classic is a sheep preaching to its flock. This was taken near Teesdale in County Durham in January 2018. I tried to take it on the move but dropped my phone and it broke. Fortunately, the photograph was salvageable. The phone was not.

Fiona continued in her email:

I normally don't do anything social on a Tuesday night because it wreaks havoc with my exercise routine and I worry about starting down the slippery slope to being lazy, but I'm really glad I did – thank you.

Fiona

PS. Last summer, on a bike tour home through Ayrshire, we saw a sheep long-jump a cattle grid.

Fiona, I'm glad I turned out on a Tuesday night in Hexham, too!

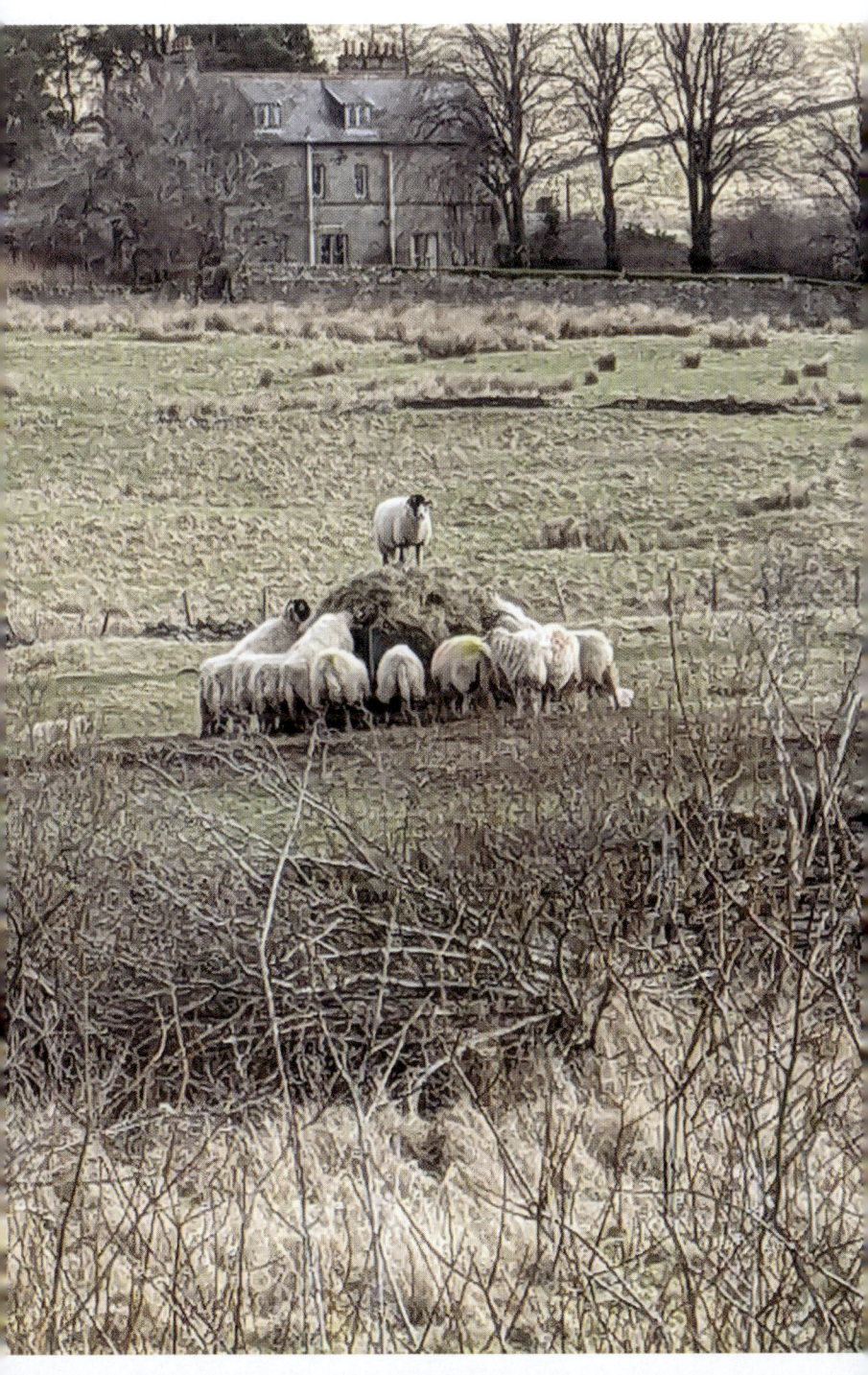

Nice People

Belle's elderly owner was so worried about her dog's health with the prospect of the major operation that was required as a matter of urgency, that tears welled up in her eyes. Molly, one of our vets, had explained everything and went through details again at the reception desk. We'd operate as soon as morning surgery had been completed. The urgency of the surgery on a Saturday afternoon underlined the seriousness of Belle's condition.

"But I don't think I can get back to collect her later on today," the lady added tearfully. "I can't drive and my friend brought me down just now. He's busy this afternoon."

Luckily, the conversation was overheard by another client sitting in the waiting room with his young son and new puppy, awaiting a vaccination. The chap recognised the lady – it transpired they used to live in the same village – and, without any hesitation, he instantly came to the rescue.

"It's fine," the man volunteered, "I can give you a lift back later. I've got a big pickup and it's no problem to come back to help."

It was shortly after this when my phone rang and I was drafted in to help too. At that moment, I was lying in the sun on a grassy bank, nursing a sore neck. I'd been enjoying the sunshine and some (semi) free time on a Saturday morning out on my mountain bike. The dry conditions made the trails fast – a bit too fast as it turned out. I'd crashed and landed on my head. The morning's adventure had been cut short by the accident. As it happened, the biking would have been truncated anyway, by Belle's illness and the need for an extra pair of hands to deal with the emergency.

"Yes, that's fine. I'll come back straight away and help," I said, "I'll be about fifteen minutes."

Belle was a middle-aged collie. Her vague illness had quickly and efficiently been diagnosed by Molly as a pyometra – a serious infection of the womb, where the organ fills up with fetid pus. Toxaemia can quickly develop so vets usually don't hang around because ovariohysterectomy is the best and most effective solution, removing the whole, pus-filled organ.

Belle was already sedated when I got to the practice and we wasted no time in getting her anaesthetised and ready. The list of consultations continued to grow, so Molly had her hands full, but I carried on with the surgery, dressed in my scrubs and cycling shorts. It must not have been a pretty sight. The distended uterus was not pretty either, but at least it was out of her abdomen before too long. She'd do well and a combination of efficient diagnosis and prompt treatment was sure to effect a full cure.

Later, Belle was up and about, seemingly not too much the worse for her surgical ordeal. Experience has taught me that dogs are usually best recovering in the loving environment that is their home, especially when the owner is anxious and worried. I arranged for her to go home, which was more complicated than usual because of three people needing to be in the same place at the same time.

"I overheard the conversation this morning and knew I could help," the kind volunteer explained. I recognised him immediately, the son of a farmer who I worked with many years ago, right at the start of my veterinary career. He was grown up now. Very grown up.

In the post-Covid, end-of-clapping-for-carers era, it's still worth remembering that not all heroes wear capes. And even if we are not all heroes, it warms the heart to realise (despite everything going on in the world) that people are nice.

Dressing Gowns

It wasn't supposed to happen at 10.30 on a Tuesday evening. But animals rarely follow the rule book. Mercedes, the little Yorkshire terrier, was not even aware of the existence of a rule book. I had palpated her abdomen and then scanned it with the ultrasound machine, five weeks earlier.

"There's a few in there, I'm sure of that," proclaimed her owner who, for the sake of anonymity and for the purposes of this story, shall be called Margaret.

"Well, I can feel and see at least three," I confirmed, suspecting that there was at least one more puppy than that inside the pregnant bitch. Over my time in practice, I've learnt that it is a dangerous game to predict the exact number of puppies. There's often at least one tucked away under the rib cage, impossible to feel or see. And good as the ultrasound machine is, it can only pick up a few foetuses on the screen at any one time, so it's not easy to tell if a baby has been scanned and counted already.

There was much excitement that little Mercedes would be a mum before long. The gestation period of a bitch is nine weeks; sixty-three days. It can fluctuate within a day or so either way but not really any more than that. Horses, by comparison, can have a pregnancy well in excess of the median figure of 340 days, (the range is 315 to 365) which makes it harder to predict the time of birth.

Margaret and her friend (and Anne and I) were therefore taken by surprise this evening and a flurry of text messages flew back and forth, flagging a problem. Mercedes was in labour a whole week early. We arranged to meet at the surgery. I estimated their travel time and the amount of organisation Anne and I would need and was pretty much spot on. Just as we'd got everything ready, the door beeped, signalling that somebody had arrived.

My eyebrows shot up in surprise at the sight of two elderly ladies shuffling into the waiting room dressed identically in cream towelling dressing gowns and fluffy slippers. I wondered if there had been a mistake. Were they looking for the spa? On closer inspection, I could see that they were weighed down by the little terrier and tackle for keeping newborn pups warm. Margaret lifted the rotund and straining patient onto the table.

"She's a fair size and she's just started pushing," Margaret explained. I examined the whelping bitch and it was clear the birth canal was open and ready, but sadly, the first pup was presented sideways, making a natural birth impossible. A caesarean section would be required. I explained what would happen next and we whisked Mercedes into theatre. The dressing-gown clad, soon-to-be-parents were left to wait.

"Can you show me where the toilets are? I've just had a water tablet," were Margaret's parting words. From here on, everything was routine. Over the years, I've lost count of all the caesarean sections I've performed. Across all species, it must be heading towards four figures. I don't perform the operation every day, of course, but one busy Saturday early in my career I did three bitch caesars on one afternoon. Busy spring days could have a couple of sheep caesars and a cow to do. I've even done one on a pig. As I dealt with Mercedes and Anne revived the babies (there were four, so my "at least three" covered it) and monitored the anaesthetic, we remarked how slick and efficient tonight's procedure had been. It was successful and uneventful, apart from the disconcerting attire of the owners. I just wish I had a suitable photo to complete the story!

Hamster in Space!

After tea on a Sunday evening is one of the few occasions in the busy week when our whole family is in the same place at the same time. We finally have time to re-live exciting moments and recount anecdotes from the past week and to discuss the challenges each of us face over the coming seven days. As well as the real-life stories, and in the same way, I suspect, that all families do these days, there is usually an exchange of amusing stories discovered on the internet via mobile phones or laptop screens. The topics come in all shapes and sizes, but the one which recently gained universal approval from the Norton family was the story behind the headline: *Hamster survives daring trip into stratosphere on flying balloon.*

Appearing on Anne's news feed, it was impossible to ignore. As she read the details of the hamster's amazing voyage into space, I expected the next bit would reveal the story had dubious journalistic origins. We can all remember a similar fanciful (and also alarming) headline involving a famous comedian and a hamster. (Freddie also had celestial connections.) But this did not prove to be the case.

Reportedly, the "world's most adorable astronaut" reached an altitude of an amazing 14 miles! Just as amazing, the little rodent is still in excellent health after his high-altitude expedition. He was recovered from his presumably deflated balloon somewhere in the sea near Japan. The video recording stopped working during the descent, so we have no idea how surprised, confused or excited his free fall might have been. This might well have been the most interesting part of the experiment.

But anyone who knows hamsters will realise that the hamster was sure to have enjoyed his foray into space. These creatures are extremely cute and I know most of them enjoy a challenge. I've witnessed this personally and professionally. Once, on my consulting room table, a peach-coloured Russian hamster swung from the roof bars of his cage in front of my very eyes, traversing the whole width of the roof like an acrobat. Was he trying to prove his health and vitality in front of the vet? I've also seen footage of hamsters running their wheels faster than Usain Bolt. Unaware of the forces of nature, in particular centripetal force, at a certain rate of knots the energetic hamster flies out at a tangent. A quick internet search of any combination of the words "hamster; fast; wheel; epic fail; funny" will bring a huge smile to anyone's face and improve a bad day.

Equally, Ardal O'Hanlon's rendition of Hammy the hamster in the classic *Tales of the Riverbank* is fantastic. It's worth a watch and even funnier than the YouTube clips of my favourite small mammal. In the film, Hammy is the main protagonist. He lives in an old boot. His friend, Roderick the rat, owns a small (obviously it's small – he's a rat) motorboat. There is a guinea pig, too, called G.P. Resourceful and creative, G.P. is an inventor and his house has a watermill. He also owns a plane and speaks in a thick Yorkshire accent. The late and great Jonny Morris OBE narrates while Stephen Fry (owl), Steve Coogan (Roderick the rat) and Jim Broadbent (G.P.) add other voices. So, as you can imagine, it has all the ingredients to make it a classic.

Interestingly, as we read on, the company who sent the hamster stratospheric is planning to repeat the trip next month, when they hope the video will work to record his facial expressions all the way back to earth. Strange times.

Collapsed Lungs

For no explicable reason, Thirsk Vets have treated two dogs with very similar, very serious and very unusual conditions. Under normal circumstances, a veterinary surgeon might see only a handful of cases of pneumothorax in a career. We've had two within the space of eight days.

Pneumothorax is the technical term for a "collapsed lung". Penetrating injuries to the chest are the usual cause, but the first case, in a young and energetic kelpie, came out of the blue. In his case, the lung had collapsed due to (we think) to a small tear developing in the delicate tissue of the respiratory system. The result, whatever the cause, is that air escapes into the space around the lung, inside the rib cage. Its proper name is a *tension pneumothorax*, because of the pressure changes within the chest cavity. The phrase always makes me smile, because "tension" also describes the atmosphere around the staff who have to deal with this emergency. The kelpie was rushed in and everyone leapt into action, hardly having time to explain the condition and its seriousness to the worried owner.

But I try not to be tense or stressed, despite the fact that affected patients are acutely ill and dangerously close to death. Panicking, I have come to realise, is not helpful in cases of crisis.

First, we need to diagnose the problem. In theory, this is simple - a dog or cat who can't breathe, is turning blue and whose heart beats are not audible by stethoscope (the thick layer of air inside the rib cage muffles the usual heart sounds, so the chest is uncharacteristically silent). If we have time, X-rays confirm the diagnosis and then a long needle or tube is inserted into the chest cavity to suck out the extraneous air. We've all seen emergency departments on television with medics shouting for chest tubes and such like. It's more or less the same in a dog, but without the shouting.

Within moments, the kelpie improved, re-inflated and depressurised.

The previously panting, blue-gummed Australian sheepdog was soon pink, wagging, breathing freely and cautiously heading home.

As he was discharged, we finally had chance to explain what had happened. The condition was termed "idiopathic", which means that we didn't really know what caused it or why it had happened.

"Oh, that's interesting," said the owner. "I had exactly the same when I was a lad." A follow-up check the next morning confirmed everything was back to normal.

The next week, our second collapsed lung was definitely NOT idiopathic – the cause was horribly evident. The hectic and unfortunate Border collie called Lucy had run into a farmyard spike and impaled herself, leaving a deep and penetrating wound on her chest. Like the boy in Amsterdam, the collie's owner held a clenched fist inside the gaping hole, preventing any more air escaping. It was *d*éjà *vu*, as I reached for the required equipment and rushed little Lucy into theatre.

I sucked about four litres of escaped air from her chest cavity. The nurse and veterinary student (who could hardly believe her luck at experiencing such a drama) watched with increasingly large grins as Lucy's breathing settled and a healthy colour returned to her previously dark purple gums. Next it was time to investigate and deal with the wound. Exploration revealed that it extended deep inside Lucy's chest and my fingers felt the unnatural sensation of the inside of the collie's ribs. I flushed and cleaned the accident zone and repaired it as closely as I could.

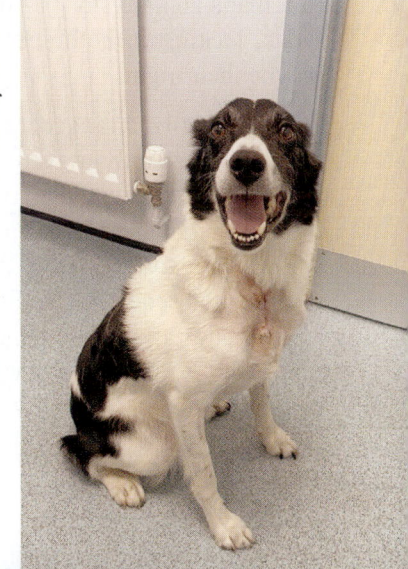

Lucy stayed hospitalised for a few days, but the wag of her tail the following morning told us everything we really needed to know. And, at last, the tension was gone.

She's Electric

I've gone green! At least, in so far as I've recently got an electric car. A combination of soaring fuel prices and the fact that there are so many EV evangelists who love their silent vehicles persuaded me to make the switch. Or even to flick the switch.

I always thought that a fleet of electric cars, with charging points in the car park would be a fantastic idea for a mixed veterinary practice. The cars could charge during afternoon surgery, while the vets squeezed anal glands and peered into dogs' ears, so would be fully energised ready for a night duty, even if the veterinary assistants were not. With most farms fairly close to the practice, even a busy work day would involve travelling no more than double-digit distances, electricity was surely the answer. Unfortunately, senior colleagues did not share my vision and my scheme never came to fruition.

Of course, electric vehicles are not new. In days of my youth, clinking bottles of milk were delivered on milk floats, silently trundling their way through the night-time streets in the small hours. Being spotted by the milkman, up late and in the garden with your girlfriend, was a sure sign you had been up to no good (but that's another story). Anyhow, I think lead-acid powered milk floats, lacking in both speed and range, have had their day. Or maybe their night.

After a hastily arranged test drive (not in a milk float), I was uncharacteristically moved to make a swift decision. I signed on the line. The car would arrive in just a couple of weeks. Plenty of time, I imagined, to have a charging point installed on the outside wall of the garage. Sadly, the information page which displayed the essential requirements for suitability for a charging point came several days after I had handed over my money for said charging point, and it turned out our garage electricity supply fell short by some distance. Also paid was the deposit for the car. Three days later, I collected the new vehicle. I asked a few final questions, including, "When does it need a service?"

There was a moment of embarrassing silence, as both sales people looked at each other.

"We don't really know. The car is very new and, to be honest, nobody knows. Don't worry, we'll tell you when we have the answer," they said, reassuringly. As my engineering student son kept saying, "The thing is, there is nothing that can go wrong with an EV." I hoped he was right. At this point I didn't have a foolproof charging method, and as I drove out of the forecourt, I had just a small niggle of concern. I could think of something very real that could go wrong: no power!

However, some very impressive work from the electrician, early on a Saturday morning, rescued my dream of having an endless fountain of energy and fuel, without having to drill too many holes in the house, much to Anne's relief.

A week later, I absolutely love my car. I have become another evangelist. It zips along smoothly and effortlessly, without noise or pollution. I feel virtuous and I almost always have a smile on my face when behind the wheel. I've completed my longest journey this evening: 92 miles. When I arrived home, the screen said I had 150 miles left and 43% of my charge. I was pleased to have traversed Yorkshire without collapsing on the hard shoulder, but was 43% remaining at the end of the day a good result? But by morning, with my new charging pod, my car, like me after a good night's sleep, should be re-energised and raring to go. I have a busy day, so I hope both the car and I will be fully charged.

Swiss Epic

I'm writing this with a sense of trepidation. Tomorrow is day four of the renowned trans-alp mountain biking race called The Swiss Epic. My eldest son, Jack, and I decided to enter on the spur of the moment, about six months ago.

"I'm looking at entering this biking race," said a friend. "It's supposed to be epic." That was pretty much all it took to persuade this father-and-son duo to click the boxes on the website. The magnitude of the adventure we were undertaking took several months to sink in, but the enormously long drive to the starting point in Arosa – probably the most isolated and remote town in Switzerland – set our nerves on edge.

We had a couple of days to acclimatise, which was lucky because stage one took us up to over 2,500 metres. There isn't much air

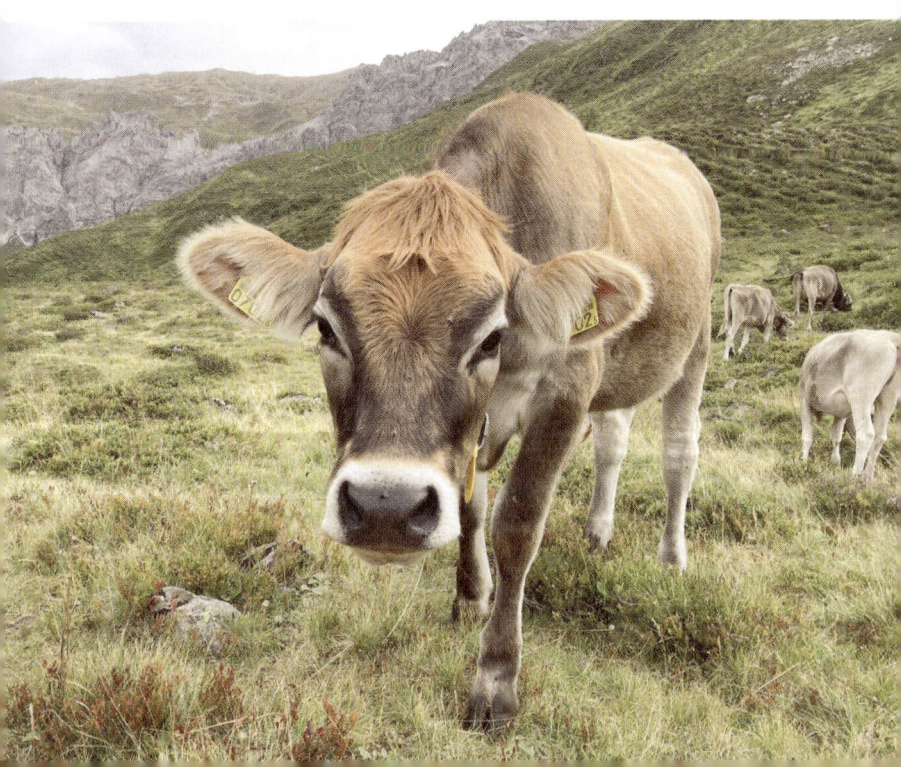

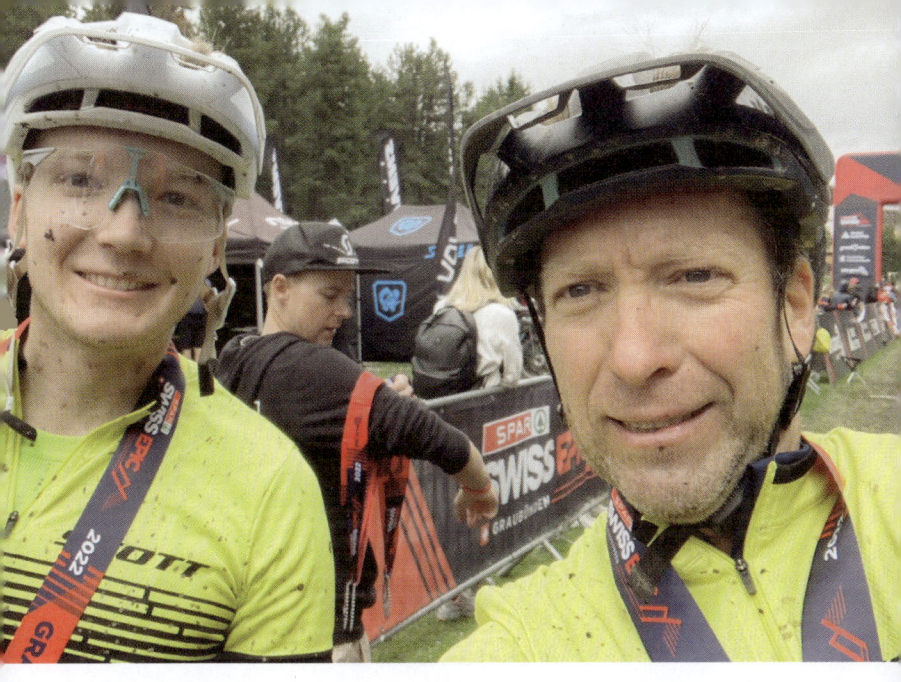

Jack and I at the end of the Swiss Epic mountain bike race, which was literally epic. This was an amazing five-day experience and it was such a joy to race with my oldest son. For most of the time I could keep up!

up there and valley dwellers like us are prone to struggle. Whilst Yorkshire has its fair share of tough climbs and challenging rides, the altitude at the top of Sutton Bank could offer no help in dealing with the depleted oxygen levels of the high Alps. A long exploratory ride around the mountains between Arosa and Davos (Europe's highest city and home of the annual World Economic Forum) proved hot and steep.

By the end of day three, Team Norton was placed in 75th position. For a team who was 50% over fifty, this wasn't too bad, especially considering over 450 teams were competing. There were competitors from South Africa, other alpine countries, the Antipodes, USA, Brazil, Colombia and everywhere in between –

we were pretty happy. Day four, though, is the hardest day. One hundred kilometres in distance and 2,800 metres of climbing. I've just had a text message from the organisers, to tell me that our starting time is 07.17.30. We need to be ready to go just 17 minutes after the elite men set off. I decided it would be a good idea to go for a massage, to improve the chances of my legs holding out. There was a special deal on for weary mountain bikers and it seemed rude not to take advantage.

You can imagine my surprise, when a rather large, bald-headed German-speaking man appeared, apparently annoyed that I was a few minutes late for my appointment. I tried to explain and apologise, but his strict voice firmly explained that, whilst he could speak perfectly in German, Italian and a language called "Franco", he was not able to speak a word of English. I nodded, sensing he did not want any conversation whilst I was on his massage table. This was possibly a good thing.

I don't often partake in professional massages, but I quickly realised that Wolfgang (as I will call him) was not the usual masseur. Maybe he had been drafted in to cope with the extra demands of so many cyclists descending on the hotel. As he grabbed each ankle in turn and pulled my legs (literally) and massaged my knees (is that right?) I began to think he was probably a baker by trade, as he flapped and bashed at my aching muscles, as if preparing dough. Or maybe he was a butcher? The enthusiasm with which he slapped reminded me of one of many comedy sketches – Morecambe and Wise or the equally funny Monty Python skit with the fish slapping dance. I chuckled at the image but this was definitely not a relaxing process and even though whale-music wafted from his small speaker, I was desperate for the experience to end. Even his Germanic pleas for me to "welax" did not make it any more pleasant. Finally, and in my view totally unnecessarily, Wolfgang massaged my fingers.

But will it work? My legs do feel renovated this evening, but tomorrow is another day…

Wild Animal Rescue

The two young children sat in the waiting room with a bucket and worried expressions. The metronomic swinging of their legs under the chairs belied their concern for the welfare of the contents of the bucket. Alf Wight, better known as James Herriot, famously advised his son Jim, at the start of his own veterinary career, to be very wary of cardboard boxes and buckets in a vet's waiting room. But the contents of this bucket were not dangerous and would not bite, scratch or cause any damage at all to the unsuspecting veterinary surgeon. Inside was a pigeon. An injured pigeon.

"We found it on the grass," said one of the two girls breathlessly. She had clearly been nominated to do the talking. "It didn't look very well so we picked it up. There was a boy there, and he asked if he could look at it. But when we showed it to him, he hit it on the head!"

I imagined this had not helped the poor pigeon, which looked confused and dazed. I couldn't help wondering if it was confused and dazed before the boy, or as a result of the boy. But it didn't really matter. I was faced with a dazed pigeon, in a bucket, rescued by two young children. Everyone involved had been traumatised by the nasty boy.

It's never easy to examine a wild bird. They are easily frightened and, unless there is something really obvious like a broken wing, they don't display illness readily. This was a young bird, still with a hint of down and a slightly bendy beak. Its eyes were spinning and its head was going round and round like a cartoon cat who had been outwitted by a cunning mouse. I agreed to hospitalise it, administer some anti-inflammatory drugs and hope that the concussion had subsided by morning.

Off went the girls, pleased the pigeon was in safe hands. They chatted excitedly as they left the practice, and were overheard by Anne as she waved them off – "That was the Yorkshire Vet, and that other vet, she was the Yorkshire Vet's wife!"

Of course, all vets have a duty of care towards any animal that they look after and should and would happily tend to an injured bird like this. But complicated cases also arise regularly. I remember, some years ago, travelling out late on a Sunday evening to capture a fox with an injured leg. It was in a bad way and the motorist had sat with the frightened fox by the side of the road until I'd finished calving a cow and eventually arrived. With thick gloves and a wire basket, I safely captured the poor animal and, before taking it back to the practice to examine, explained that I would treat the injuries if I could and then release it back to the same wooded area as soon as possible. But if the injuries were too severe, I'd humanely euthanise the fox.

I was surprised by the emotional reaction of wailing and tears as soon as I'd said this.

"But why won't you repair the leg if it's broken?" protested the Samaritan.

I tried to explain that it was often not appropriate to perform surgery on a wild animal, especially where a lengthy recuperation period might be required. It is simply too stressful for the animal and, more often than not, it is the stress of close human contact that kills them rather than their injuries. Minimal intervention is key to successful treatment.

However, as I injected the pigeon in the bucket, I felt sure that my simple treatment would save the pigeon and save the day!

Swallows on the Wire

The swallows have lined up on the wires ready for their long journey south. I hope they have all enjoyed their summer holidays in the north and that they have had their fill of Yorkshire bugs, enough to sustain them for the trip.

Signs from nature like this – along with the ripening of berries and the falling of apples – tell us that summer is over and autumn is on its way. For a mixed practice vet, there is a brief respite. Over most of my career, I've noticed that September, for a vet, has been the quietest month of the year. It might be because cattle are still outside, ruminating on the last nutritious swathes of grass. Later on, it stops growing and loses any useful nutrition, and the inevitable wetness means that the cows need to be brought indoors, to save the fields from becoming damagingly churned up and muddy. The rush for summer vaccinations for dogs and cats has subsided – holidays are now over and fewer animals need kennels or catteries. Also, summer seasonal allergies subside for dogs, so the waiting room is sometimes as quiet as the autumnal stillness and misty mornings outside. In a few weeks, cold and damp will develop, and pneumonia can quickly become a serious problem for young cattle. As October and November arrive, vets become very busy again. Autumn-calving herds start to require assistance, along with the usual jobs that come with housing stock.

But despite the brief lull, at the onset of autumn and the end of summer some odd illnesses can prevail. Harvest mites – tiny fluorescent orange bugs – appear at the end of august and early September every year. They can cause havoc for sensitive cats and dogs, but are ephemeral little blighters and soon disappear as September progresses. Fog Fever is an aptly named respiratory illness that affects cattle grazing in September. A wide-bladed grass called *Yorkshire Fog* loves the autumn conditions and thrives. In susceptible cattle, a molecule in the grass can cause Fog Fever. It sounds like a disease from medieval England although modern science can explain the pathogenesis of the illness. Strange fungal diseases appear too – Rye Grass Staggers is a peculiar condition which I've only seen once. A small herd of heifers fell victim to this weird disease and developed strange locomotion. At least one of them wandered along walking backwards!

For farm-animal vets, it's the time of year when the countdown for pregnancy-testing beef suckler herds begins. Hundreds of cows will return from the moors and meadows to winter housing shortly. They've been running with a bull for two months or more, testing his stamina. In a few weeks' time, it will be the stamina and strength of the right arm of the vet that is tested as each one in turn is checked for pregnancy. High up on the edge of the moors, for many back-to-back years, I knew a tough week was waiting. Three hundred cows belonging to one farm needed to be pregnancy-tested. These cattle had barely seen a human being for the whole summer and were usually in a bad mood. Partly because they didn't want to be inside a cow shed, partly because they didn't want to be separated from their calves and partly because they were not expecting to have an arm inserted into their rectum. Kicks and violent objections were frequent, and escapes were common. The whole process, which included weaning and moving from farm to farm, took three long days. After each long, cold day, I would count myself lucky to have avoided injury and sometimes hypothermia. At least my right arm was warm for most of the day!

Smelly Cat

"There's a gentleman on the phone saying his cat smells," reported a rather surprised Sue as she emerged from behind reception. "He doesn't know why. He can't work out where the smell is coming from."

The cat was duly booked in for a check-over. It reminded me of some wise words I once heard from an RSPCA vet on a BBC television series about vets, many years ago. A dog owner complained of a similar problem. As a veterinary trainee, I'd occasionally dip into this programme, in the hope of gleaning some useful tips. I can remember clearly the vet explaining that the smell might be coming from "His ears [a case of otitis]; his mouth-[stomatitis or halitosis]; his skin [dermatitis]; or his anal area [there is no veterinary terminology for this smell]". Obviously, there are various smelly conditions which can emanate from this region. The vet then calmly examined each body part, carefully checking, and then sniffing, each area of the increasingly confused patient. Sadly, I don't remember the eventual diagnosis. On reflection, the world of the "TV vet" has changed considerably since those days.

The case of the smelly cat also brought back more recent memories. Late one evening, at a practice where I used to work, a colleague was called to check over another "smelly cat".

"He's started to smell. So, we decided to give him a bath in the kitchen sink, but it hasn't really made any difference," explained the owners as they unloaded the cat from its box onto his consulting room table. Bizarrely, the cat was stiff as well as smelly and had evidently been deceased for some time, *rigor mortis* having set in. My colleague, according to his detailed clinical notes, carefully listened to the chest before confirming the obvious. What was less obvious, was whether the cat had died before or after its dunking in the kitchen sink. Was it smelly because it was dead or dead because it was smelly? We'll never know the answer to this riddle. I'll leave readers to speculate.

Later in my working week, I had another unusual experience. It didn't involve any smelly animals. I was summoned to London for an appointment with a pile of almost one thousand books. Each one requiring my signature. My latest book, *Adventures with a Yorkshire Vet: Lambing Time and Other Animal Tales*, is out on 6th October. It's an illustrated book, aimed at younger readers. I've received my complimentary ten copies already – an author's perk – and, I have to say, the book looks lovely. The black and white line drawings are exceptional (thank you Jo Weaver), evocative and realistic.

I've signed many books over the last few years – more than I could ever have imagined – but never so many all at once. I remember fondly the very first one, which I did with trepidation, under the supervision of Sue at White Rose Book Café in Thirsk – the venue for each book launch.

"No, you need to sign it on the title page," Sue explained. I knew nothing about title pages and remarked that I should be able to sign it wherever I liked: it was my book after all! But I followed her instructions and every book since I've inscribed on the right page.

The staff at Walker Books were experienced in the process of bulk-signing and organised an efficient system, spare pens and an endless supply of strong cups of coffee. Three hours later, there was just a handful of books left and I had writer's cramp and blurry eyes. It was worth it though and, happily for everyone, by book number seven, I'd achieved another publishing goal – a book with a front cover *without* my face on!

RDA

Last Tuesday I spent the afternoon at a golf course just north of Leeds. I don't often frequent fairways, and I couldn't remember the last time I had been anywhere near the eighteenth hole. Apart from the ones on mini/crazy golf courses, of course. But I was not clutching a club. Instead, I was talking to the large crowd assembled to raise funds for a the Stockeld Park RDA (Riding for the Disabled Association).

After a contact several years ago, a lady called Pam had invited me along. "We had Amanda Owen a few years ago and it was very popular," she explained, trying her best to encourage another writer/Yorkshire-based TV character to address the audience. Immediately, I was keen to help. My first experience with Riding for the Disabled was as a student, when I spent some time with a fantastic vet called Mark Collins. He was a whirling dervish of energy, knowledge and experience and I learnt a huge amount during my time at his York practice. In the middle of a characteristically jam-packed day, he explained that the next visit was "very special". It was an RDA centre and Mark explained how all the work he did there was free of charge. "The work they do is so important," he added.

I can't recall exactly what Mark was doing with the horses that day, but I do remember seeing the joy on everyone's faces as horses walked calmly around the arena; the demeanour and spirits of each rider were lifted immeasurably as soon as they got onto their steed. It seemed the horses realised they needed to be especially careful, and the experience was gloriously positive for everyone. Last Tuesday, as I chatted to Pam and some of her friends, she explained that there was a constant requirement for volunteers, to enable this amazing organisation to continue. Each horse and rider needed three assistants: one to lead and one on either side to steady the child atop and help with balance and confidence.

I gleaned more information during the afternoon. This group began in 1973, with the aim of providing riding lessons for children with special needs around Harrogate and Wetherby. Originally, the base was Stockeld Park but is now at Harrogate Riding Centre. Currently, twenty-four children benefit from the experience, improving balance, posture and communication skills. Not least, it's also a lot of fun! There are no charges made for the sessions, so the costs are covered by fundraising; which is where I came in this afternoon. The room was packed so I hoped we'd raise plenty of funds. I also hoped I would remember what I had planned to say. I looked down at my hastily written notes, which were supposed to give me prompts for each of the topics I wanted to cover and anecdotes connected to each one. Unfortunately, I have terrible handwriting. Most of the important words had been written down too hastily and my scrawl was almost illegible, even to the author of the words. I put the notes to one side and prepared to ad lib for forty-five minutes. I need not have worried. The audience were kindly attentive and amused for the most part. By the end, I felt sure I had earned my sandwiches and cuppa!

Later, I learned some good news: my afternoon talk-and-tea had raised sufficient funds to cover riding lessons for thirty-two children. That means thirty-two smiles and thirty-two confidence-and-balance-boosting sessions.

The sessions happen every Tuesday during school term times and extra volunteers are always required. If you can spare a couple of hours on a Tuesday and want to make a big difference, check their website: www.stockeldparkrda.co.uk or drop Pam a message on 07908159901.

Ambushed by a Cat

A poorly lurcher was on its way down as an extra appointment. Over the phone, the case sounded serious and urgent and not something that could wait. Even a fully booked consulting list can accommodate a proper emergency. We'd fit him in.

When he arrived, Ed looked very sorry for himself. A placid lurcher can look lugubrious at the best of times, but the Harry Potter-like gash in his forehead was deep and painful. It seemed to make Ed's ears droop even more than usual and he looked as confused and bewildered as he was sore.

"He's been ambushed by a cat!" explained his owner, indignantly.

"Oh dear," I replied. "I don't think it usually happens that way round!"

"It's a great big ginger tom. He'd been hiding in a bush, waiting to pounce. I watched the attack from a distance but there was nothing I could do. He dived on poor Ed when he went past," recounted Ed's mum, before adding, "He's a real menace around the village!"

Images of cartoon cats and mice came to mind, where a different Tom was usually the perpetrator of violence as well as the victim. I wondered if this tom had planned to use a heavy metal object and if a pointy, throbbing lump might appear on the dog's head as stars and tweeting birds circled.

Once upon a time, the hierarchy was clear. In my childhood, my grandparents' garden was filled with Jack Russell and Bedlington terriers along with their own lurchers. Woe betide any feline who was fearless or foolish enough to venture nearby. Then, *all* dogs chased cats (and rabbits); cats chased mice; birds ate insects (although I do know an old lady who swallowed a fly. I'm not sure what happened to her). Now, the old lines seem to have blurred. The times, as Mr Dylan once said, they are a changing. I know many cats which happily cohabit with dogs. I even know a goat called Abbie that hangs out with the farm dogs. "She thinks she's a dog," explained the farmer once upon a time. And I know a pig which lives in a kitchen, happily sharing a bed with two Labradors and a three-legged huskie. In our own household, on a sunny day, our hapless but happy rabbit hops and jumps in the garden with Emmy, our Jack Russell, for company. They seem to be friends, although the harmony of the relationship is really based on mutual ignoring rather than shared interests. But any friendship between a terrier and a lop would have been implausible in times gone by.

But back to the unfortunate Ed. On closer inspection, there was no throbbing bulge on the top of his head nor circling stars. Just the zig-zag laceration, like an attack from the foil of Zorro, bisecting Ed's forehead almost perfectly. It was deep but clean and most of the earlier bleeding had stopped, but it definitely needed some stitches.

After some light sedation, a neat clip and a clean, I instilled some local anaesthetic and carefully placed a row of sutures. Surgery like this is very satisfying and not at all stressful or too challenging. When the edges are re-apposed, the pain quickly dissipates and healing can begin. Ed looked much better as soon as he came round (he didn't even seem to have an Ed-ache) and we summoned his owner back.

"Come back in ten days for those sutures to be removed," I instructed as I handed him over, with a couple of bottles of medication. "And, whatever you do, Ed, keep out of trouble and stay away from the bush. Remember, it's an Am-bush!" Nobody, especially Ed, appreciated my joke.

Head in a Watering Can

We've had some cute patients this week. Clifford was the first. A kitten, just a few weeks old and covered in ticks. His rescuer brought him in to see us, enveloped in a towel. With his head popping out of the top, as he surveyed the scene in our prep room, he resembled a fajita – expertly folded so that no bits of kitten could escape. It was an impressive piece of wrapping and, held aloft for the obligatory photos of every cute patient, Clifford looked like Simba from *The Lion King*. Immediately, we were smitten by the kitten. But there was nothing wild about the feral, so it was a simple, though painstaking, job to twist off each horrible tick one by one. These ugly parasites seem to be more and more common. They attach, then suck blood until they become engorged, then fall off to lay eggs and perpetuate their life cycle.

Only two days later, Clive appeared and his owner was quite upset. Clive was a puppy who had developed the exciting habit of sticking his head into the watering can. There was obviously something interesting at the bottom of the can, but best of all (I imagine) was the noise that Clive could make with his head inside the metal container. This hobby was funny and fine whilst Clive was five or six weeks old. His head was small enough to fit in and pull out without incident. But it was Saturday when disaster struck. His head had grown but the can had not. The unfortunate pup careered round the garden, bashing into bushes, trees and garden furniture. After several minutes, Clive started to panic and so did his owner. Eventually, the puppy's head was prised free, but the sharp metal rim of the watering can had torn his ear. Blood was oozing from the prominent gash. It needed to be cleaned and sutured so we arranged an emergency appointment. The jagged cut was deep but simple to repair once the sedation had kicked in. Fresh wounds heal quickly.

As Clive recovered from the ordeal, his owner admired the neat sutures. We chatted about the habit that animals sometimes have of inserting their heads into things. My own, first puppy had a penchant for putting plant pots on his head. Watching a four-month-old Border terrier running around with such headwear is probably one of the funniest and most joyful sights I can remember. And my gosh, he really *was* a cute puppy. I've seen more than one cat come into the surgery wearing a full-sized tin can, much like a medieval knight about to enter a jousting competition. The taste and smell inside the dregs of tins of tuna are too much for a cat to resist. Thankfully this is not too common but, amazingly, most cats wear such head gear with remarkable calm, despite being plunged into perpetual tuna-infused darkness. A colleague once reported seeing a cat with a jam jar on its head. It was challenging to remove but at least the cat could see out!

But the funniest of all is surely a heifer wearing a bucket. In every herd of cattle there is at least one troublemaker. Like the school classroom clown, an attention-seeking bovine can work out how to flip the handle upwards in just the right way and at just the right time to make a spectacle. Whilst undertaking a TB test some years ago, I watched a young Friesian heifer, calmly walking round the fold yard with an upturned yellow plastic bucket looped over her ears. Unlike Clive, she showed not a trace of panic, and the herd instinct kept her safe.

"I hope Clive has learnt his lesson," said his owner. "Maybe I should introduce him to plant pots or buckets rather than watering cans!"

Well Oiled

I knew the day would be a challenge as soon as the bloodhounds arrived. It wasn't so much that the two saggy, drooling canine super sleuths were a problem per se, it was that both had been doused liberally in baby oil. As they slid into the waiting room, a dangerously slippery trail was left in their wake.

"They've been badly affected by fleas," their owner declared, adding with confidence, "And this works really well. The little buggers don't stay on for long!"

"I'm not surprised! They probably just slip right off," I replied, as I examined each dog before its operation. I tried to explain that modern ectoparasiticides are extremely effective as well as safe, and don't bring with them the health and safety issues associated with an excessively lubricated floor. But my explanation fell on deaf ears as I took the slippery pair into the kennels. They slid into the walk-in kennel together, specifically designed for large dogs. Today, it felt appropriate to change the name from "walk-in" kennel to "slide-in kennel".

The glistening surface of both dogs acted as an interesting topic for discussion, especially for other staff members who had not been involved when they arrived at the practice. They did not necessarily know the story. I could recount a similar tale, of an occasion when I was just as lubricated as these hounds. It was some years ago, at the start of my very first triathlon. I stood confidently in a grassy field on a damp day in June near Lake Coniston in Cumbria. I had squeezed into a wetsuit, which left little to the imagination. In preparation for the event, some weeks earlier, I'd been urged by my friend and enthusiastic coach to "cover myself in baby oil". It would apparently "make it [my wetsuit] easier to remove once I'd exited the water." Somehow, these instructions must have got lost in translation, because all the other competitors looked similar to one another, their suits matt black like a wiped blackboard, while I was slick and shiny. Apart from looking like a total idiot, my oily surface presented a dangerous risk to aquatic birds as an oil slick was left in my wake. As I wrote this article and recollected that day, I tried to remember the year. I asked Anne. She swiftly found a photo of me standing in a field, under a charcoal grey sky, wearing an orange swimming hat that made me look like a Kinder egg, and a glistening black wetsuit as shiny as patent leather shoes. It was my first triathlon and I'd only recently learnt how to swim over arm. The swim was frightening because the water was cold, deep and black. "I remember that day," I say with wistful nostalgia.

With a loud guffaw, Anne says, "So do I!"

Thankfully, there was no loss of birdlife on my account after the Coniston Mountain Triathlon all those years ago. And fortunately, despite the slicks around the kennel area, prep room, corridors and waiting room, nobody slipped and broke anything in the aftermath of the bloodhounds.

Later, as I discharged the patients, I discussed with the owner how the surgeries had gone and followed up with various post-op instructions, one of which was not to drench the poor dogs with oil again. The ridiculous scenario was made worse as she explained that she'd administered the very same treatment to every dog in her very large menagerie. The fleas had been eradicated (I suspect they slid to a neighbour's house) but there was another, unexpected consequence.

"They must think I'm weird in my local shop," she said. "I've been going through five bottles of baby oil every week!"

Skippy

I've spent many years helping with rescue and rehoming charities and have seen first-hand the many challenges that face those committed to this worthy vocation. One of the less stressful elements though, is thinking of novel names for each animal that passes through. In the nineties, characters from *Friends* provided a reasonably rich vein of names for rescues. Back then, there were hundreds of cats called Chandler. Nowadays, UK prime ministers, or even cabinet members, would give an almost endless supply – though how this would do for their chances of gaining a loving home is anyone's guess. But for the little kitten brought into the practice today, it was an easy task to pick a name.

The tiny kitten, no more than a few weeks old, had been found in a skip. Finding kittens is, apparently, an occupational hazard for the local skip hire company. As well as extra refuse from neighbours with bursting wheelie bins, they frequently find abandoned kittens in their skips, which is awful. This tabby and white tom seemed very pleased to have been rescued from his metallic prison.

"This is Skippy," said Lucy, as she introduced him to me, excited to have saved the day. "We've called him Skippy because he was found in a skip. It's a good name, don't you think?"

I did think the name was apt and I also agreed the kitten was cute. I went to say hello, and Skippy meowed in the high-pitched and wide-mouthed way that only happy kittens can. Later that day, during a gap in my afternoon consultations, I went back to make better acquaintance. Skippy, after a big meal, was now fast asleep in a warm and comfortable bed. I didn't feel like disturbing him.

Back in the 1990s, every similar kitten would routinely have been blood-sampled for the troublesome viral twosome of FIV (Feline Immunodeficiency Virus) and FeLV (Feline Leukaemia Virus). These viruses were prevalent in many feral kittens and had spilled over into the domestic cat population. Nowadays, largely thanks to a highly efficacious vaccine, FeLV is very rarely diagnosed. I can't remember the last time I saw such a case over recent years. A sole case of FIV the other week (a feral cat found in a barn) made everyone's head turn. Once upon a time, positive cats would be a daily occurrence.

It reminded me of my early days in practice and as a student, when soon-to-be-retired senior vets would puff on their pipes and rub their chins at an unusual canine patient. "Could it be a case of distemper?" Any dog with a peculiar illness could have distemper ascribed as the diagnosis, its variable signs ranging from a cough, diarrhoea, crusty nose, hard pads or neurological disease. Old vets could apparently hear distemper dogs coming down the corridor, their solid and hyper-keratinised pads making a distinctive clicking noise. Of course, and again thanks to the development of a robust vaccine, distemper has pretty much been eradicated. Certainly, I have never seen a case in my thirty years connected with veterinary practice. This is a good thing.

Another disease, thankfully consigned to the history books and the memory of older vets and farmers, is Brucellosis. Once endemic, this disease caused abortion and swollen udders in cattle and intermittent (undulant) fever, sweating, back pain and crippling depression in humans. Naturally, people exposed to cattle were at increased risk and Brucella infection was blamed for the melancholy of many farmers and vets of the last generation. It was testing and culling (and the arrival of Foot and Mouth Disease in 2001) which finally sent this nasty disease packing, rather than vaccination.

The battle against infectious disease is a long one with many twists and turns.

Goodbye Brucella, Hello Other Diseases

Last week, I touched on the happy decline in cases of Feline Leukaemia Virus over the last few decades. In 2022, in contrast to how it had been in 1992, it didn't cross my mind to perform a viral test on little Skippy, the cat found in a skip. (Incidentally, and just as happily, Skippy has found a new home, with walls and a roof, comfy sofas and kind humans, rather than metal and full of rubbish.)

Other animal diseases have also disappeared over the same period. BSE came quickly and out of the blue but was eradicated very slowly and at a great cost. In my view, it was nothing short of a miracle that the British cattle farming industry survived that mysterious disease. Foot and Mouth Disease (FMD) appeared with equal speed, caused havoc, then disappeared in almost as miraculous a fashion. Eventually, it seemed there were just not enough cattle and sheep left alive in the UK to allow transmission of the acutely infectious virus. Ironically, the mass cull of cattle in 2001 to try to control the Foot and Mouth Disease outbreak had a bonus effect on another disease: it was the final nail in the coffin of Brucellosis. The biennial blood and milk testing of every breeding bovine over two years old had seen the number of cases fall steadily during the 1990s. But, in the aftermath of FMD, brucellosis disappeared too.

Still in the cattle world, TB has a perennial presence. The perfunctory testing, if we are honest, has totally failed to control this slow-burning disease. There is not sufficient space here to cover the ins and outs of this problem and nor am I sufficiently qualified.

So, to the latest infectious disease crisis. Bird flu has no easy answers or solutions. I'm certain that the road signs on grass verges around the country declaring *animal disease control zone* provide neither. As I look up and see actual birds flying above, none of which can read the signs, the measures seem even less useful than the disinfectant-soaked pieces of carpet that covered lanes and farm tracks in March 2001. Poultry farmers can keep their birds indoors for ever, but as long as wild birds can fly, an infectious disease affecting our feathered friends will surely never be controlled in this way. It was just the same when we humans were instructed to stand two metres (or was it one and a half metres?) away from each other whilst queuing outside the supermarket. Or even inside the supermarket, for that matter.

Meanwhile, birds become sick, test positive, get culled or die. Baby puffins (pufflings) are found dead in heartbreaking piles on the Farne Islands and gannett numbers decline at Bempton. Someone told me yesterday, as we chatted whilst his dog became sedated sufficiently to be safely examined, that it's impossible to buy duck breasts anymore. While we can all probably manage without duck breasts, Christmas is on the horizon and the spectre of no turkey will seem unbearable for some. The same person who told me about the duck situation also advised, "If you see a turkey anywhere, just buy it. I reckon there won't be any in the run-up to Christmas."

My mind went back to equally fraught times when another disease rampaged with positive test results and death. The shortage that time was, mercifully, not turkeys, but toilet paper. Inexplicably, given that the disease caused coughing rather than diarrhoea, sensible, fully grown adults could be seen in droves with armfuls of toilet paper. All without any shame or embarrassment. I wonder what the pre-Christmas rush on turkeys might look like!

Encouraging Kids to Read

This week, I headed to Lancashire. On a specially arranged day off, I traversed the A59 with a car boot full of books and some trepidation. My destination was the Ribble Valley and a village called Read. This was a coincidence, because encouraging children to read was one of the reasons for my visit to Red Rose country. I was going to Read, in both senses of the word.

Some weeks ago, Katherine, a teacher at the village primary school, contacted me to see if I would come along to talk to her pupils, with my new children's book. Although this was outside both my locality and my comfort zone, I felt compelled to find time. Katherine's enthusiasm was hard to refuse, as she explained that it was becoming particularly challenging to find ways of encouraging youngsters to pick up a book, rather than an iPad, phone or games console. The effects of lockdowns and Covid had exacerbated the insidious decline in reading, she told me. Katherine thought that a visit from a vet off the telly, with boxes of books aimed at younger readers would be a great stimulus.

This was the third such event that I'd attended in just over a week. In the planning phase, I'd wondered how I could capture the attention of my audience, many of whom, I felt certain, would have no clue who I was (I thought this was especially likely when speaking to a Lancastrian audience). The production team of *The Yorkshire Vet* very kindly compiled a selection of clips from the programme to give the kids a feel for what they might have missed on a Tuesday evening, after bedtime for some. There was the fail-safe mix of new life, different animals, lots of slime and poo, amusing noises and images of cows breaking wind and puppies who had eaten party poppers. The final clip had so far had everyone in stitches when a baby alpaca toppled over like an AT-AT walker in a Star Wars film, after I had applied splints to her front legs, inadvertently using bandages that stuck to one another as she tried to walk.

This having captivated the audience I was off to a flying start. "Does anyone here think they might like to become a vet?" I asked. A multitude of hands shot up. I spoke about the challenges and joys of my career and more recently of being able to take part in making a popular television series and about becoming a writer. I read out a short section from the book. This has always been my least favourite part. I hated reading out passages from books or Shakespearean plays at school and from my own book, well, it just seems like showing off! But proper authors and book retailers assure me that it is *very* important.

With fifteen minutes to go until the dinner bell, I was drawing to a close, "Has anyone got any questions?" Again, hands shot up from all over the hall. The questions covered everything, from how to get into vet school (from the older kids) to "What has been your most challenging case?" and "What's the funniest animal name you have come across?"

Handing out copies of the book to all the kids of the appropriate age, I thought my trip across the Pennines had been very worthwhile. These young people had wisdom and maturity in abundance and way ahead of their years. I hoped they would enjoy my stories and that at least some might develop a further interest in a career with animals. If not, then at least some might have been encouraged to read. I was really pleased that *I* had been encouraged to Read too! Thank you, Katherine.

Dogs on Tables?

"And I have one more question," said a dog owner after I'd finished listening to Arthur's heart, checking his healed wound and administering a vaccination. "When did vets stop putting dogs on the table?"

I was taken aback – it was not the usual question at this point in proceedings. I sprang from the floor and re-assumed my earlier and more familiar position, half-leaning against the units in the room, near the computer. "That's a good question," I replied and paused for longer than normal before answering. The pause was kindly interrupted by my interlocutor, "Because in the olden days, vets would *always* insist on dogs being on the table, no matter how large or small."

She was right. I thought back to the days when I was a keen sixteen-year-old. I would spend Thursday evenings at my local practice in Castleford after school. The senior vets would never have dreamt of scrambling around on the floor after an anxious dog, no matter what size they were. As my veterinary career has progressed, I have lost count of the number of pairs of trousers which have been consigned to the bin because of holey knees, so much time has been spent on the floor. It's better for nervous dogs, for sure – when do dogs ever get put on a table under normal circumstances? It's no wonder they sometimes get worried.

The discussion continued to cover the evolution of other veterinary habits.

"And I know you used to wear a tie for work. You don't anymore," came next. A statement rather than a question. I agreed and explained the circumstances which prevailed decades ago. Young vets would be sent home if they dared to come to work without a collar and tie. Now, polo shirts embroidered with a logo, or scrub tops (à la "American Hospital Drama") are more common attire. I have to say, it's more suitable, especially when rummaging around on the floor. I spent some time in America, working in a veterinary ER. Everyone wore scrubs suits and even went out for lunch in them. I thought that was odd. It was like going out for a burger dressed in your pyjamas.

"When I first started work, I used to wear a white coat," I added, "and a brown one on farms."

White, "lab" coats were common for doctors, vets, lab technicians and pharmacists. They had useful pockets for equipment but, for a veterinarian, this was the limit of their practical benefits. White coats quickly became grubby around dirty dogs, in contrast to the clinically pristine environment in a laboratory or a surgery devoid of animals. The brown coats for farm work, just like those worn by handymen or staff working in hardware shops, were even less practical. They lacked any proper protection from farmyard semi-solids, were difficult to wash and took three weeks to dry. Waterproof plastics have long-since superseded this antediluvian outerwear.

Later that day, I examined a golden retriever with a sore leg. She was immediately, and without request from me or second thought from her elderly owner, lifted up onto the table. After the examination, I recalled my earlier discussion about dogs-on-tables and the changing habits, which had been noted.

"Well, it's easier to examine her if she's on the table, isn't it?" said the owner, matter-of-factly, before adding, "Maybe it's that vets are getting younger. Maybe they can bend down and stand up again more easily than the old vets. Maybe that's why more dogs are examined on the floor."

He made a good point and could easily have been correct. I called in my next patient, Fluffy. She was a cat and not as benign as her name suggested. Despite still not feeling like an "old" vet, and perfectly capable of bending down and standing up again, I would definitely not be examining her on the floor!

Emmy in the Wars

My Jack Russell terrier has been in the wars recently. A visitor to the house was playing games with her and unknowingly threw a stick into the garden for her to chase, unaware of the dangers. Emmy was equally unaware and, charging after it with typical enthusiasm, grabbed it, but not without accident. It was not her usual tennis ball and a high-pitched squeak immediately alerted the humans to a problem. Luckily, with two vets on hand immediately, the cause was readily identified – an inch-long laceration under her tongue, bleeding and sore.

These injuries can be very nasty, especially if the puncture extends deeply, if a piece of the twig snaps off and becomes embedded, or if the penetration occurs amongst the important structures at the back of the throat. It is especially bad if the injury is not spotted straight away, for example if the squeak is not heard. Emmy – and the mortified guest – were both lucky. The laceration was not too deep, quickly spotted and relatively simple to fix. The hardest bit was looking into her dark eyes as the anaesthetic agent trickled into her vein to send her to sleep. Exploration and then flushing with saline and antibiotic solution left the laceration clean. A neat row of dissolvable sutures finished the job. She would soon be back to normal.

I know how painful these injuries can be. One Sunday morning, when on call, a belligerent horse did not want a deep cut on its front leg to be sutured and, with speed and accuracy, kicked me in the face, driving my teeth through the inside of my lower lip. It swelled up almost immediately with a horrible stinging pain. For some reason, once I'd returned home to lick my wounds, I decided the best thing to eat would be something soft, so set about making myself a mountain of mashed potato. I'd heard that this sort of thing would help. It did nothing of the sort and there was more searing pain as each starchy mouthful stuck to the damaged tissue. There is still a thickened scar at the site of injury. I think the mashed potato was a bad idea. I didn't offer any to the dog today.

But Emmy's enthusiasm is as legendary as it is carefree. Once, she spent a full afternoon playing a ball game with my little nephew, Luke. As we watched from indoors, it was hard to tell which of the two was having more fun. Luke wasn't that good with his aim, and the ball kept going into the bushes. Each time an increasingly dishevelled Emmy would appear, ball in mouth and shrubbery in her coat, but wagging her tail with glee. Anne went out to suggest it might be time to end the game. Emmy was exhausted and it was only a matter of time before she sustained an injury. But the herbaceous border had already sustained injury, almost beyond repair. Bushes were flattened and battered, flowers had their heads knocked off and even the lawn was worse for wear, with scuffs and divots as if a rugby match had just finished.

"I think we should have a break, Luke," came wise and cautionary words from the kitchen door. "Or maybe try to keep the ball on the grass?"

"But it's absolutely fine," declared Luke, with the authority and confidence that can only come from a four-year-old. "If I throw it into the bushes she just goes in and gets it!"

Back to this week, and she's made a full and complete recovery from the recent injury. Lessons have been learnt and our visitor has promised it will be balls only from now on. As for Emmy, she can't make any promises to stay out of scrapes.

Trainees

We have plenty of trainees at the moment, which is a very good thing. They include new veterinary graduates, working in their first job and learning the ropes; nurses undertaking college training courses; wannabe vets working during a gap year before university; and students helping out, cleaning kennels, wiping tables and tidying up so they gain some invaluable insight into the veterinary world. At last count, we had eight students of one form or other, between the practices in Thirsk and Wetherby. Next week, for one day only, I'll be supervising, advising and overseeing the most interesting Herriot trainee of them all. But more of that later.

Watching and trying to guide a reticent youngster as they find their way through the veterinary maze, negotiating their way through mistakes and navigating challenges, is an uplifting and exciting journey. It reminds me of my own early days. They say you learn from your mistakes. That must make me as wise as an owl. Leaning in too closely to a dog's backside, to get a better view of the process of "emptying the anal glands", was one early mistake I'll never forget. My face and hair were splattered by the eruption of foul-smelling, fetid anal gland contents. A similar thing happened with a male ferret, which necessitated a total change of clothes. I'll not make either mistake again!

There was the time, during a pre-vet school placement at a practice near the Dales, when I was given the task of replenishing the empty bottle of thick brown antiseptic. The vets used it for cleaning everything before obstetrical procedures. I'd cleaned out and tidied up the lambing pen after the vet had finished, and rummaged under the sink, searching for the viscous liquid, so that all would be ready for the next patient. Each of the big, brown bottles looked similar. Later, a red-faced (and brown-armed) and very annoyed vet emerged from the next lambing, calling angrily, "Which idiot filled the antiseptic bottle with floor cleaner?" It was an easy mistake to make, I told myself, especially for a trainee!

In earlier times still, after school and at the vet's in Castleford, I had the job of putting tablets in pots. I know now that this is a very important job, that requires a second set of eyes to double-check everything is correct. Back then, a weary sixteen-year-old was deemed to be a suitably qualified and capable person, but when an owner returned with her still-coughing cat, it became clear I had made a big error.

"I've done my very best to get Daisy to take her tablets," she said despairingly, "but she just can't seem to swallow them." To my horror, I realised that I'd dispensed dog-sized tablets rather than tiny ones suitable for a feline. That time, it was me with the red face.

Happily, our current crop of students and aspiring vets and nurses seem to be much more capable, and I look forward to watching their progress. Over the years, I've lost count of all the newly graduated veterinary surgeons that have arrived brimming with enthusiasm, some like rabbits in the headlights, then steadily developed confidence and untold capability. Many of my early colleagues have gone on to make the profession proud. Even Ben, whose standard advice for any gastro-intestinal irregularity was to "feed plenty of moist, green vegetables."

Now, with two new and growing practices, we too are proud to be able to help and encourage new blood and new enthusiasm into our profession. Young people are where the future lies. Us oldies can only carry on for so long. The future, as ever, is in the hands of the next generation. And from what I can see, with our support, that future is in very good hands.

A Herriot Trainee

Last week, I talked about apprentices, students, wannabe vets and trainees. It's been a pleasure watching their capabilities increase; as well as seeing careers develop over the years. But recently, we had a totally different trainee. He arrived on the train and appeared at our practice in Thirsk with a thirst for knowledge. As I met him and shook his hand outside our front door, I couldn't suppress an enormous smile, because this guy was, quite literally, a Herriot trainee. It is a phrase I have heard many times over recent years, mostly on Tuesday evenings at 8 p.m. But Nick was the actual modern-day personification of Mr Herriot.

Of course, this vet-to-be was Nick Ralph, the wonderfully talented actor who has found recent fame in Channel 5's remake of *All Creatures Great and Small*. He plays James Herriot. In the first episode of series one, James (or Nick) gets off a bus (not a train) to find his way to Darrowby (aka Thirsk). Today, though, Nick was going to spend the day with a real-life vet (me) and I hoped to give him a small glimpse into today's veterinary world.

Nick would possibly be helping but definitely learning something. He plays a vet, but isn't one. He gives an excellent interpretation of a vet at work, just as Christopher Timothy did in the 1970s and 80s, inspiring a generation to enter the profession. And yet, as I explained how to place a catheter, induce anaesthesia, and insert an endo-tracheal tube, I was discombobulated. *He should know these things*, I kept thinking, *He's a vet. I've seen him on telly, being a vet and doing these things.*

In theatre, the surgery we were carrying out could not have been more simple. The lump to be removed was small, well-circumscribed and benign. It was a straightforward procedure and, for a real vet'nary, devoid of drama or stress. Perfect. Nick opened the packets for me as instructed, lifted the right lids off suture reels and inserted the rectal thermometer to check the patient's temperature, with skill. *Had he done this before?* I wondered.

During the surgery, I quizzed Nick about his actual veterinary experiences, on set and in preparation for filming. Flatteringly, he admitted to watching various episodes of *The Yorkshire Vet* for reference and research. The irony, and cyclicity, amused me. A vet friend, Andy, who I saw practice with when I was a veterinary student, was the veterinary advisor for the programme and had offered him tips in preparation and supervised some of the scenes.

"Obviously, we can't do procedures on real animals," Nick explained. "So we have prosthetic creatures put in place for when I have to roll up my sleeves and get my hand in!"

This explained how he managed to calve a cow without getting his shirt dirty.

"There's much more blood, slime and s@*t whenever I calve a cow," I laughed. "And you should take your top off. That's what I always do because it saves washing so many shirts – I'm sure you've got the physique to pull it off," I added, cheekily.

Later in the afternoon, much like in Herriot's tales, it was time for clinics. Secretly, I wished for a Thirsk local explaining his dog was "womiting". "He's womiting real bad, Mr 'erriot." But there was no womiting dog, not even one that was vomiting. No cases of "flop bot" and not even a deceased budgie.

But at least I managed to encourage Nick into action. He would discharge the dog whose lump I'd removed earlier.

"Mr Herriot has done a grand job," I explained to the confused owner.

Conference Season

For a few days the other week, we were in London. And I mean all of us. At least, all the Nortons. Archie was racing for his school at the Olympic Aquatics Centre in the national schools swimming finals, Jack was racing on the Thames in his university boat and Anne and I were topping up our knowledge at a two-day veterinary conference. Of course, there were old vet friends to meet up with too! In the run-up, it was difficult to determine which of us was more excited. For my part, I couldn't get over the serendipity of the three events occurring together. I dusted off my map of the Tube, before realising that new lines, over and under-ground, had been created since my ancient booklet was printed. I would need to rely on Anne's superior knowledge of the London Transport system if we were all to be in the right places at the right times.

Anne and I arrived without incident. The trains from Thirsk to London can be superb and we arrived at Kings Cross a mere two hours after dropping Emmy off at the kennels. It wasn't long before we were ensconced at the ExCel. There were more lectures than it was possible to attend, everything from *Clinical implications of new understanding of the regulation of phosphate homeostasis in cats* to *The Pale Patient*. And pretty much everything in between.

As well as some excellent lectures, there were the trade stands. All the major players, along with some newcomers, displayed their wares. Established equipment and drugs were on show, all trying to persuade delegates that one was better or more cost-effective than its competitor. More exciting were the new products and inventions. Many were captivating – like the new system for making bespoke, 3D-printed lower limb supports for dogs and cats with slack joints. The innovative design looked amazing. Had I been sitting on the panel of a veterinary *Dragon's Den*, I would definitely have been "in". The novel light therapy (which looked like a powerful torch) had a fantastic sales pitch, with some bright-orange safety goggles and a neon display, but demanded more vigorous scrutiny. The light had been shown to cure all manner of stubborn skin ailments. It reminded me of *Jamie and the Magic Torch* because it seemed very much like magic to me!

Within two productive days, Anne and I managed to catch up with old friends and reminisce over times past. We'd had some interesting conversations with some of the wise within our profession. We had collected two large bags of free pens, booklets and logo-labelled notepads as well as enjoying some lovely hospitality courtesy of the drug companies. I think we had both learnt some new and useful things and benefited from the most up-to-date knowledge. But there is no such thing as a free lunch. After some debate by text message with colleagues, we managed to spend several thousand pounds purchasing two brand-new, state-of-the-art anaesthetic monitoring machines. Oh, the colours, the smooth, aesthetically pleasing touchscreens! Not to mention the added confidence surgeons and nurses will have using such fantastic equipment! I can't wait to get them both in action.

With conference concluded, we headed to watch our sons competing both on and in the water. Against the best competition in the country, I can happily report that we had a 9th and 10th place. On the Tube back to Kings Cross, we both agreed this was more impressive than any of the vet stuff we'd seen, but we were lucky to have filled three days so completely. The final challenge – would the train be running, or would there be a delay or a strike? But the story of the train home is another one altogether…

Toilet Dog

"My Border collie fell in the toilet last week," was an unexpected final sentence in an email I received recently. The Border collie's owner had been reading one of my columns, in which an animal had suffered a misfortune. I can't remember whether it was the cut in Emmy's mouth (from which she has made a full recovery, by the way) or the puppy who got his head stuck in a watering can (who is also fine), but whatever it was had clearly moved her to tell me about this unfortunate incident. Sadly, there were no other details, so I am none the wiser and left with more questions than answers. Why? How? Is she alright? Is this a common occurrence? I've seen and helped with animals stuck in all sorts of places over my veterinary career – cows in rivers, horses in ditches, a heifer stranded one evening, legs akimbo, on a little footbridge in Sowerby Flatts – but I'd never heard of a dog in a toilet.

As another year – turbulent for many – comes to a close, it is a good time to reflect; to question old habits, appraise routines that have become the norm and set new goals for the next twelve months and beyond. The dog-in-toilet email helped to remind me that there are at least a few Yorkshire folk who read, digest and possibly even enjoy the 630-word weekly summary of my veterinary experiences. This is a comfort and a pleasure because, late on a dark Sunday evening, as I tap away on my laptop at the kitchen table, first trying to think of a topic, and then trying to sculpt it into some sort of form, nothing is further from my mind than who might actually read it. Nor what anyone might think (which sometimes comes back to bite me). I know the collie owner must have been reading it, so that's at least one. Today, on the occasion of my 300th column here, there is more pause for thought.

At a lunch meeting the other day, an old friend revealed himself as another reader of my column – confirming that there are at least two of you! As I ordered a second helping of lunch in Kofi and Co. in Wetherby last Monday, he explained all.

"I'm not really a country person," he admitted. "I'm from the middle of Wakefield, but now I live in the wild, open countryside of West Yorkshire. When I open *Country Week* I finally feel like a *real* country person!

"I pour my coffee, open the paper at page three and start reading. Then, I tuck into my scrambled eggs. I read it all, but I always start with your column." It sounded like a halcyon moment to be savoured, with all the ingredients of a perfect, relaxing morning. He went on to comment on his favourite other parts of the paper. Maybe a similar thing was occurring in hundreds of homes across our county? I hoped so.

And we have another fan. She has never opened the paper over her scrambled eggs though. Martha lives in California and fastidiously and enthusiastically subscribes to *The Yorkshire Post* online. She can access our words across the pond. Martha occasionally sends correspondence to my practice in Thirsk, full of news from California: droughts earlier in the summer, welcome recent rain, and snow high above in the Colorado hills, which will provide water reserves for next year, along with updates on her recently acquired pug called Pretzel (who accidentally ate a bee). We have an eclectic bunch of readers, that's for sure, and it's fascinating to have an insight into their worlds. Even if one of them involves a dog in a toilet.

Six Dinner Sid? No Dinners Brian

There is a children's book called *Six Dinner Sid*. It's the story of a sleek black cat who is very greedy. He visits all six houses in the street where he lives (Aristotle Street), where each resident thinks they are the sole owner of the cat. The neighbourhood is cat-friendly, but not so human-friendly (presumably everyone is busy), so nobody realises Sid is living with anyone else.

One day, Sid is poorly. He's duly taken to see the vet by one of the residents, where his temperature is taken and a bottle of foul-tasting medicine prescribed. The next day, an identical sleek black cat is presented to the vet who is surprised to see another sleek black cat with a very similar illness. The next day, you can guess what happened. Six Dinner Sid had been rumbled.

Ever since I read this story to my kids about sixteen years ago, I've been waiting to experience a real-life Sid situation. Nowadays, bigger issues exist, such as client confidentiality – the clinical details of a patient cannot be discussed with anyone other than the registered owner, let alone everyone in the street! As for the heinous mis-prescribing of six times the amount of medicine, now, frantic phone calls to the Veterinary Poisons Advice Line to confirm safe or dangerous levels of the medicine would be required; followed by a call to our insurers.

A while back, Anne came home with her own version of the story. She had been treating a cat for various issues, necessitating some blood samples and an intravenous drip. Happily, his condition improved and he was duly sent home. A few days later, the practice received a phone call from a somewhat perturbed owner reporting that their cat, having been missing for many months, had turned up with hair clipped off its front leg. Looking at the address, Anne realised what had happened, but this is where client confidentiality poses a problem. Attempting to be sufficiently vague, she managed to suggest that the cat might have been living with someone else.

At first, this was met with annoyance, but as the conversation progressed and the person on the end of the phone realised that there was the possibility of ongoing veterinary involvement (and therefore cost), a rapid U-turn was made. They decided that it was absolutely fine if their cat had decided to move house!

And then last week, I finally saw my own Six Dinner Sid, except that the cat was called Brian. He was old, thin and not as greedy as Sid. One day, the tabby was unceremoniously bundled into a basket and brought to the practice.

"He's old now and he's struggling to eat. I think there is something wrong with his mouth," explained the owner. Or at least, one of his owners, although we didn't know this at the time. Sure enough, there were huge crunchy concretions of calculus all over the poor cat's back teeth. The owner went home to look in their diary to find a suitable time for Brian to come in for an anaesthetic to sort out the problem.

The very next day, the same tabby appeared, just as thin and with the same terrible teeth. Luckily, the mystery was much more quickly solved than Sid's. The second "owner" was straight-talking from the start.

"This is Brian. He's the village cat. We all look after him. I think his mouth is sore."

"Yes, he was in yesterday," I explained. "I think he's booked in for a dental on Monday!"

It remained to be seen which of Brian's owners would get the job of bringing Brian on Monday morning, but I hoped the villagers had better communication than those in Aristotle Street! I suggested a WhatsApp group.

Jamie and the Magic Torch?

There is a new and modern piece of equipment at our practice in Thirsk. Its arrival has been met with excitement but also some scepticism. When I first heard about this new light treatment for indolent and obstinate skin lesions, it sounded too good to be true. I read the papers, analysed the data and listened to the comments of eminent dermatologists. Each of these went some way to mitigate my concerns. That said, over the years I have seen many flashy promotional pitches from drug companies, embellished with impressive graphs which collapse under scrutiny. I'm a firm believer that a genuinely good product will prove itself over time. In this case, it seemed we were one of the first to try it out.

There have been a number of these "breakthrough" products during my time in veterinary practice. The first was back in the 90s, when a miraculous new antibiotic for curing calves of pneumonia appeared. Previously moribund cattle would rise like Lazarus after an injection of just a couple of millilitres of this elixir, called Micotil. The fact that it could cause heart attacks or limbs to fall off if accidentally injected into humans added to its mystery. That some older farmers would mispronounce the drug as "micro-kill" added to its aura. The latest generation of ectoparasiticides bring another seismic shift, in my opinion – highly efficacious and extremely safe. And as for the new monoclonal antibodies that counteract joint pain in stiff geriatric dogs and cats, they are nothing short of wonder-drugs. They have improved and extended the lives of so many pets previously struggling along on a combination of anti-inflammatories and fortitude.

All of these have earned their place as excellent drugs. So, for Anne and me, as we prepared our first patient for this novel therapy, mixed up the clear gel and orange potion (aka chromophore gel), put on our goggles and fired up the gun, it was a step into the unknown. I felt like Jamie, from *Jamie and the Magic Torch*. Anne applied the now-orange gel then fired the bright blue light at the dog. This was when we realised the importance of the special goggles.

Two treatments of two minutes each with a minute in between. It was simple. Seth, the stoic Labrador, patient number one, looked the same afterwards as he did prior to the torch treatment. His swollen lower limbs were just as ulcerated and sore afterwards as before, but obviously, results weren't going to be instantaneous. The leggy Great Dane who came to us all the way from near Doncaster was next. We could almost imagine an immediate improvement.

The regime demanded a follow-up zapping a week later. Today, I've seen both dogs again. Of course, I checked the photos taken before the first treatment and compared them to today, asking the requisite question: *How is he getting on?*

"Much better" was the reply from both. The improvement was hard to deny, and it seemed like the early stages of our novel therapy had been efficacious. The theory of the coloured gel, refracting light into different wavelengths seemed to have worked. Blue light killed bacteria and reduced microbe-induced epidermal inflammation, whereas green modified dermal fibroblasts. Other colours did other things, just as miraculous.

I still maintain a healthy scepticism, but the proof of the pudding is that both dogs are coming back next week for a third zapping. On telly, I'd seen Siegfried Farnon work his magic using pluming purple powder and smoke to mesmerise a horse owner. Was this treatment along similar lines? Or was this new light therapy shining the way forward for skin disease? As always, time will tell, but it's looking good so far...

I Am the Walrus

The North Sea coast had an unusual visitor recently. His name was Thor and he was a walrus. Following a visit to Hampshire at the start of December he swam to Scarborough. Nobody seemed to know why he was visiting the United Kingdom, although there was speculation that he had heard the New Year's Eve celebrations on the Yorkshire coast were spectacular. If that was his real intention, Thor was to be sorely disappointed, because the festivities were cancelled in his honour, so as not to frighten him. Of course, this was a very good idea, as was the police cordon to keep excited spectators at a distance. Locals had enjoyed the entertainment of a visiting walrus anyway, so nobody minded.

Normally, walruses live in the shallow waters of the Arctic and sub-Arctic, typically along the eastern coast of Greenland, between Alaska and Eastern Russia, and around Northern Canada. This was the first one ever to have visited the UK. They are distinctive because of their huge bulk – a bit like Jabba the Hutt – and their imposing curved tusks. They are not generally dangerous or threatening. Their only natural predators are orca whales and polar bears, which might explain why Thor seemed so relaxed and content as he reclined on the jetty at Scarborough harbour. He was safely away from either. Appealing as Thor was though, nobody wanted him to get too comfy or outstay his welcome. Last summer, another walrus with a wanderlust found herself in a spot of bother. Freya became overfriendly and developed the habit of climbing onto the decks of small boats to sunbathe, on the fjords around Oslo. The safety-conscious Norwegians decided to euthanise the interloper, which seemed a bit draconian; poor Freya.

Fortunately, Thor's sojourn was shorter. He only stopped long enough in Scarborough for a bag of chips and some crab sticks, then he was off on his travels again, slipping back out to sea, quietly quitting the harbour walls. Destination Blyth. Maybe the nightlife was better there?

I love stories like Thor. Was he lost, or was he simply travelling the world? On his gap year, perhaps? Anthropomorphising human feelings onto (or into) animals, however, is usually not at all helpful (walruses, of course, don't have a gap year, for example) and can lead to incorrect decisions being made or wrong conclusions being drawn. We don't know what animals can think – we probably never will. However, I think it is sometimes fair to make sensible extrapolations. When I watch gangs of young lambs charging around the grassy fields in warm sunshine (it won't be long now), chasing, playing, jumping and skipping; or an eventer with adrenalin coursing through its veins and straining every sinew; or my own dog, Emmy, as she dives with abandon into the beck to retrieve her tennis ball, it's impossible not to imagine happy thoughts flooding through the minds of these creatures. Even the peaceful chewing of a ruminating cow exudes a calm contentment. Anyone who observes animals will recognise these traits and agree that happy animals are all alike. I read somewhere recently that bees enjoy playing football. Maybe I've misinterpreted that. I'm sure I read they *could play* football; I don't suppose that means they necessarily enjoy it. But why not.

As Thor made his way to Blyth and beyond, it is surely fair to assume he is having a good time exploring the world outside his comfort zone. I hope he makes his way home safely – there is sure to be a tracker following his progress, so it would be nice to keep in touch. Perhaps he'll come back to visit again one day. If he does, let's hope he pre-books his tickets to the Sea Life Centre. Pre-booking is essential, Thor. Though you might even get a free ticket.

Five Poorly Mice

The appointment booked in on my list for later in the afternoon was unusual – *Five poorly mice*. Without wanting to trivialise the illness of these little creatures, I quickly amended the line to add some more detail – *Three of them blind.*

Each time I clicked on the diary screen of the computer, I chuckled to myself and hummed to the tune of the nursery rhyme. My mirth was tempered with slight anxiety, because I couldn't imagine what might be the problem with five poorly mice. Vets very rarely get to examine mice – I couldn't remember the last time I'd treated one. I remembered the first I'd seen, many years ago. I could feel its tiny heart beating, so fast that it had a trill thrill, way too fast to count. Mice don't often go wrong, and their short life span of just a couple of years are two reasons for the non-attendance of mice at a vet clinic. Of course, they are very difficult to examine, mainly because they are so small. I hoped the "Thirsk Five" would be simple.

Eventually, three small boxes appeared in the waiting room. They rested neatly on the owner's knee. It was mouse-time.

In the consulting room, the lids were removed and five rapidly moving, inquisitive faces popped out to say hello. There were two pairs in one box with the poorliest in a box on its own, to reduce the risk of any infection transferring to its little mates.

"They are sneezing and one has stopped eating," the mouse owner explained. This sounded bad, but at least the diagnosis was simple. I plugged my stethoscope into my ears and attempted to listen to the chest noises of the worst mouse. It was impossible to make any proper assessment, but evidently they had a respiratory infection. I've treated many rats with the same conditions and reached for the most effective drug – a long-acting antibiotic, perfect for respiratory infections. There was a palpable sense of relief on the mouse owner's face when she realised there would be no need for oral dosing. I just had to calculate the micro dose and inject the stuff. Diluting the medicine down was like an A-level chemistry exam, but it went to plan.

Later that evening, back at home, I donned my cycling attire and headed to the gloom of the garage to my training bike. This is a hibernal habit of many enthusiastic cyclists who strive to maintain sanity and fitness during the dark and cold months. Over the years, I've discovered that it is essential to change quickly and not get too warm or comfy indoors. After a long day at work, even vacillating for long enough for a cup of tea can put the kibosh on an evening training session. Despite the barren interior of my garage, I can quickly become immersed in podcasts, Netflix or even a colourful, virtual world full of other virtual cyclists on glowing virtual bicycles, ascending virtual hills and passes. The cyber-magic means that other cyclists – in their own garages and sweating into their own patch of salty concrete floor, slowly disintegrating as a result of sweat-induced erosion – can be travelling up the same virtual hills. Somewhere near the top of Mont Ventoux, I caught a glimpse of something most definitely not virtual. Its legs moved faster than any of the virtual cyclists and it was brown and small and furry. It was another mouse. The sixth of the day. Just as I spotted him, he spotted me and stopped his scurrying and turned to stand on his back legs, staring straight at me. He looked very curious, quite healthy and fat – probably, judging by the nibbled bag, from eating my rabbit's food and also the foam of my yellow paddleboarding shoes. For sure, the healthiest mouse of the day.

Wimba Way!

Like buses (but unlike trains), we've had two novel therapies arrive in close succession. The first, recounted recently in this column, was a new treatment using a bright blue light and an orange chromophore gel. It seems to be helping improve indolent skin conditions and the successes continue to add up. The second was just as exciting but before I got to use it, a virtual meeting was required. I've not had a Zoom meeting for some time, now normal meetings are deemed safe. However, in some circumstances, the huge savings in both time and travel make a Zoom event appealing, if not essential. On Friday, my virtual companion was on the far side of Europe – Poland, in fact – so a real meeting was virtually impossible.

Maciej and I were discussing the new invention developed by his company. The product is called "Wimba" and its techniques, I'm told, are based on the twin modern miracles of 3D printing and "Augmented Reality". Maciej's company promise to analyse measurements and video clips of the lower limb of a lame dog and create a bespoke orthotic support, specific to the dog's defective limb. The first tranche of development is aimed at helping to support a nasty problem called "carpal hyperextension". This is where the wrist (the joint in the front leg above the foot) extends more than it should, because of slack ligamentous support behind the carpal joint. It's a horrible condition in which dogs have near constant pain and shift the weight intermittently from one foot to the other, like a guilty school boy in front of the headmaster. The surgical correction is serious and involved, with a lengthy recovery, so any option to avoid this will be good.

As soon as I met the people from the new company at a conference a month ago, I knew they were onto a winner.

"At first, we focus on the carpal joint," the MD explained personably. "But we aim to make supports for other joints. And also, shoes. Hard ones for town and soft ones for the countryside." It sounded like all avenues had been explored and options covered.

"What a brilliant idea," I effused. Before long, we'd exchanged email details, a package had arrived with the equipment and said Zoom meeting had been fixed up.

I had a candidate in mind and, Zoom over, called her owner, hoping she would be a willing first volunteer.

"How is Willow getting on?" I asked. She was coping OK, although some days she didn't want to go for a walk. She was happier to lie on the sofa. I explained the invention and the process and we arranged an appointment to investigate. I showed Willow's owner the videos and photos and arranged the little motorised buggy, as I had been instructed. I explained that, with my mobile phone attached and set in video-mode, the buggy would complete a circumnavigation of Willow's lower limb, recording the angles and nuances of her lower leg. She'd wear a tight-fitting sock, a bit like a snug version of a leg warmer to smooth out rugosities caused by a hairy leg. Once recorded, this video would wing its way to Poland, where a perfectly fitting support would be created and sent back to Thirsk.

Would the Wimba way work? As I set off the little robot, gamely clutching my mobile phone, I marvelled at such amazing innovation. All the time I couldn't get a tune out of my head. It seemed incongruous and yet apt at the same time.

In the jungle the quiet jungle, the lion sleeps tonight. A Wimba way, a wimba way...

I hoped the Wimba way would work.

Special Patients

Frank the Labrador-cross-Staffy had only been in the practice for an hour or so but the mark he made was indelible. The paralysis of his vocal cords, the tell-tale dribbling of urine and the suspicious knuckling of his front leg bore all the hallmarks of a progressive neurological disease. The prognosis was grave. Despite the seriousness of Frank's illness, his happiness and joyful character spilled out in abundance. He played with his blanket, tugging at its edges and rolling over before hiding his face under its cover whilst lying on his back. As the diagnosis developed and the prognosis became undeniable, we all took turns to sit with him, fussing his ears and keeping him cheerful up to the end. At the end, later that day, he brought his ball with him. Everyone cried. I felt awful, because earlier I had confidently assured him, "Don't worry, old boy, we'll get you right." Not for the first time, my optimism was misplaced and I was sadly wrong.

By way of mutual consolation and to lift the gloomy mood, we all chatted later about how some patients find a special place in the hearts and memories of practice staff. Usually, this is because of a long-standing battle against illness, or a protracted recovery from difficult surgery, typically fought with a stoic cheerfulness and a wagging tail. Sometimes it's a rare condition that we've diagnosed when other practices had not managed. This makes the resolution all the more satisfying. Winston the bulldog had seen many vets by the time he got to us and he was in a pickle. He has a rare autoimmune disease called *Pemphigus vulgaris*, (which is as nasty as it sounds), but now we have sorted out his treatment and when he comes for his fortnightly check-ups, Winston's presence in the waiting room cheers everyone up. His persistently wiggling body and snuffling happy face provide an infectious source of delight. Winston is a star.

Nurse Lucy told us about one of her favourite patients in a previous job. He had become the practice cat. A chronic skin condition led to the obvious moniker of "Scabby", but a diagnosis of diabetes meant his owners couldn't cope with the management and expense, so Scabby moved into the vet's. He lived in the cat kennels by night and frequented Pudsey bus station by day, scrounging morsels of fish from the chippy or attempting to grab a free bus ride.

"He was a lovely cat, and a real character," remembered Lucy. "He used to sit by the PDQ machine and swipe his claws when clients tried to pay!"

One of my most memorable cases, and best canine friends, was a Border collie called Bobby. It took me months to diagnose his rare illness, including several lengthy discussions to eminent pathologists, one of whom was in America. Bobby came in every week for treatment and for me to take blood samples which eventually confirmed the problem. Even though he invariably felt awful, and must have been sick of my needles, he would wag his tail and lift up his front leg for me to take yet another sample or instil another intravenous injection. His bone marrow failed in a cyclic pattern, so once every three weeks, Bobby's white blood cells would drop dangerously low. This left him prone to bacterial sepsis, in the same way as a chemotherapy patient. On occasions, I'd visit Bobby at home and he'd always show off by charging round the garden at high speed. I tried a number of therapies, which worked for a time and up to a point, but, in the end, the outcome was inevitable. Needless to say, when the final injection came and Bobby's tail wagged for the last time, there were tears in abundance.

Vets in the Community

Last Wednesday I headed out of the practice, south down the M1 and out of the county. My appointment was with a charitable organisation at a Nottingham vet school called "Vets in the Community". This wonderful, student-led organisation provides basic care for the dogs (and cats) of homeless and vulnerable people in Nottingham. I've been involved since pre-Covid times and had promised that I'd go and see what they were up to and hopefully help as soon as I was able.

A mobile caravan, jam-packed with bandages, stethoscopes and basic drugs visits two parks on alternate Wednesdays and offers an open-air open surgery. By the time I arrived a queue had already formed, and the whiteboard displayed details of broken nails, coughs and scabby skin. Students worked in pairs to ask questions and perform the necessary examination.

I asked if this was scheduled into the students' clinical rota as part of the curriculum.

"No, it's volunteers only," they explained. "It's better that way. We have to select the students each week, from all the different stages."

I chatted to some of the dog owners, all of whom expressed huge gratitude for the work of the volunteers. Most grateful was the chap who had a coughing and spluttering Staffie. "This dog means everything to me," he explained; its eyeballs bulged with each paroxysm. I hoped we could find out the problem and help. Of course, with only basic facilities, pragmatism would be king. "I should be in my element," I thought.

It wasn't long before I was called in to help with the scabby cat, as the students came to report their findings and conclusions to a clinician. Even though my knowledge level was far below that of the university veterinarians, I immediately felt at home, having seen thousands of such cases over my career – probably more than the highly qualified experts, who would rarely see the run-of-the-

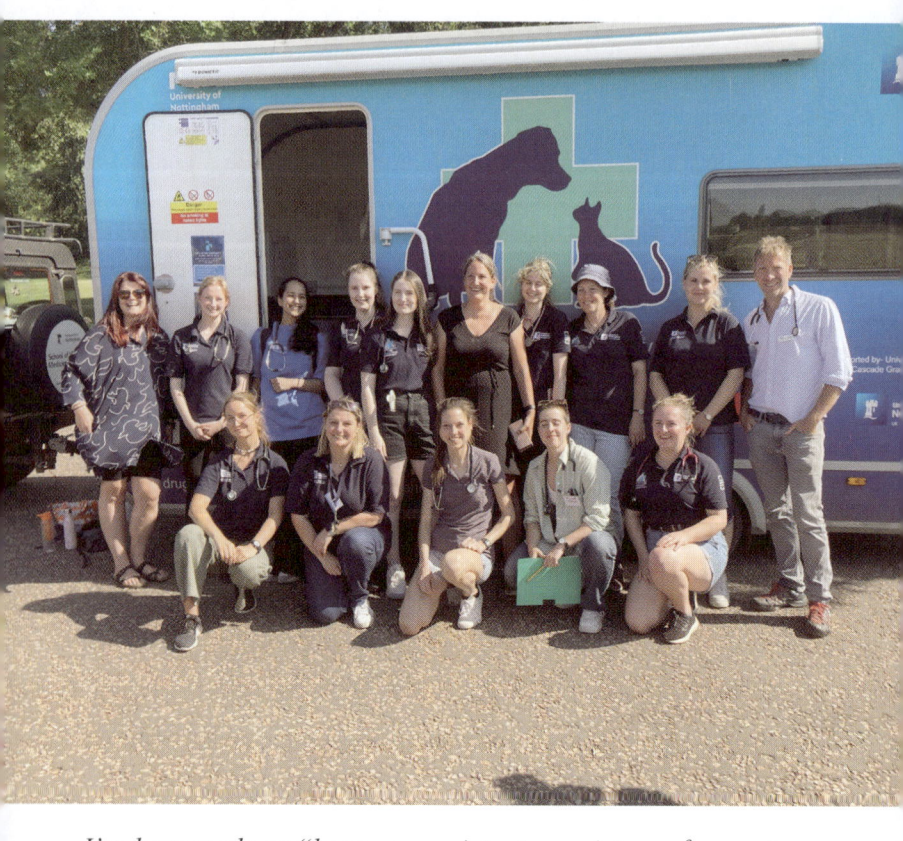

I've been made an "honorary assistant associate professor at Nottingham vet school and I help (as often as I can, which isn't often enough) with their charity work helping the animals of homeless people in the city.

mill, first-opinion problems that we see all the time in general practice.

"Can you describe the lesions?" I asked the most senior looking student. My question surprised him. He was obviously looking for guidance on the diagnosis and treatment.

I went on, "It's really important to be able to describe the problem, so that another vet (or soon-to-be-vet) can compare the situation when the cat comes back for a follow-up." Before long we had all the right words in the correct order. "Diffuse, extensive, raised, exudative, erythematous, scaling with some alopecia and pruritis."

"So, what's the diagnosis?" Blank faces. Eventually, we'd agreed on *miliary dermatitis*, a common cause of intractable itching with scabs on a cat. It's often caused by flea allergy. I added some extra information, which I can still remember being told by my bushy-bearded pathology lecturer at vet school, and which acts as an *aide memoire*.

"It gets the name because it feels like millet seeds have been sprinkled into the cat's coat." There were more blank faces. I suspect millet seeds are not a typical part of a student's diet these days (though to be fair, they weren't in those days either). We talked about the treatment options and I sent them off to calculate a dose of the appropriate medicine – a long-acting steroid injection, which works like magic. We scoured the caravan for a bottle of the stuff, but to no avail. The scabby cat would need to take tablets. I made a mental note to bring a few bottles of essentials and some syringes next time I came to help.

Aside from the occasional blank expressions on my trainees' faces, I was incredibly impressed by the organisation, commitment and capability of these young veterinarians. From what I've seen, the animals of the homeless in Nottingham and the future of our profession are in excellent hands. Even if nobody has heard of a millet seed.

Shagging in the Pub

After a cold, dark and frosty mountain bike ride, my mates and I were all delighted to get to the safety and warmth of the pub. As the fatigue sets in, the "beer tractor beam" seems to get stronger. Night riding is exciting and, enveloped by darkness, all the emotions are heightened. Some people – most people, actually – think it is a crazy idea and a foolhardy pastime. It probably is. But with friends and powerful lights, a mountain bike ride in the dark is more thrilling than anything I can think of that is legal. Arriving at the pub, where a log fire will be burning warmly and a beer will be waiting, makes for a perfect end to the evening.

Our ride started with a short road section, followed by a stiff climb up to the top of Kepwick Bank. Under a moonless sky, frosty grass and heather and icy puddles glittered in front of our lights. Then we headed into the woods and onto some twisting single track. It was a fast pace but punctuated by stops so everyone could catch up. The final steep, rocky descent was one I'd completely many times before in daylight. I knew the position of every boulder and the smoothest and fasted line was etched in my mind. But somehow, with bright lights and shadows, wild animals and eerie noises, it was like I was riding the trail for the first time. Before long, we were flagging. Some of us had low batteries, with torches flashing weakly rather than providing unlimited lumens. Others had cold fingers, frozen feet or exhausted thighs. I regaled my riding companions with Herriot-style tales of calving cows in the nearby fields, or treating sheep with impossible prolapses in the fold yards of farms we rode past, as a distraction, but everyone was pleased when the lights of the pub came into view, glowing in the distance. We packed away the bikes and changed the muddiest of our clothes, ready to plonk our weary bodies on a warm and comfy bench. As my colleagues opened bags of crisps and supped deeply on pints of strong lager, I had other things to ponder. Red, the little rusty coloured pub terrier, immediately recognised me. He'd had an appointment with me the previous week. His enthusiastic hormone-driven humping had been putting some of the customers off their pints. On one occasion, he even caused a spillage on the carpet. My job was to anaesthetise him and remove the cause of this problem. It went smoothly and Red appeared to hold no grudges over my intervention.

He rushed up to me with a customary wide grin and wagging tail.

"He seems very pleased to see you," commented a fellow drinker who had a smart shirt and a mud-free face.

"Yes, it's surprising," I replied, "because last time he saw me, I had just removed his testicles. Luckily, I don't think he's made the connection!"

I settled myself onto a comfortable cushion on the fireside bench and eyed up the frothy glass in front of me. I'd earned this and raised the glass to my ready lips and closed my eyes. Just then, I sensed a presence on my left. The small terrier had leapt beside me. He stared deeply into my eyes, then wrapped both his front legs around the upper part of my arm and gave it a grippy hug before embarking on a rapid rhythmic thrusting which almost made me spill my drink. I steered him off and onto the floor, but Red was still determined.

Though irksome, I could smile because I knew it would only be a matter of time before the hormones subsided and Red's misplaced libido became a thing of the past.

Taxi Deliveroo

I'd just popped into town to try to book a table at our local Italian for the following night. I felt sure the popular restaurant, which is in the former NatWest Bank (look it up, it's really worth a visit), would already be booked up. I hoped that by turning up in person, I could persuade the manager to spare one of his precious tables. Of course, he could. Good restaurant owners know how to attract and keep customers.

After my successful booking, I dropped into the nearby off licence to grab a bottle for the evening. An old friend appeared as I was perusing the bottles of red. Marcus was once a fearsome fast bowler and Botham-like batsman and one of the best cricketers in the area, partly because of his immense skill, but mainly because of his enthusiastic leadership on the pitch. Playing for Bagby village, I can recall memorable victories at Sharow and Markington, with Marcus opening the bowling and batting at number three. But his biggest claim to fame, at least as far as I was concerned, was his prowess as a cowman on a local dairy farm.

He worked as cowman for a herd just outside Thirsk at the time when my veterinary career had just started. What he didn't know about cows was not worth knowing and I used every opportunity when visiting the farm where he worked to glean extra bits of practical knowledge. I had a thorough theoretical grasp of facts, medication regimes and illnesses of all types, but like many nascent vets, it was perfecting the practicalities that I craved the most. "For cystic cows, I allus reckon you can't beat a PRID," he'd say and new-vet-me would take mental note. He'd have top tips for fixing blocked teats – techniques that you'd never find in a textbook, and persuasive ways to coerce a cow into an AI cubicle. In the shop this evening, it was great to catch up briefly and we reminisced over past times and previous bovine ailments.

In front of the spirits section, he pronounced proudly, "I once gave a cow a whole bottle of whisky just like that one. She had eaten too much kale and an old vet from a practice in Wetherby where I used to work said the only thing that would help was a bottle of whisky, so I poured a whole one down her throat."

"And did it help?" I asked.

"No. She died immediately."

Nowadays, Marcus's cricketing and farming days are over, but he throws himself with the same enthusiasm into his new job and has a thriving taxi business.

"I need the cheapest bottle of wine," he explained to me and the man behind the counter.

"Are you not working tonight?" I asked.

"I am, yes. But this is a delivery. Someone's called me to pick up a cheap bottle of wine and deliver it to her house."

Times have certainly changed. Local village cricket is pretty much a thing of the past, largely consigned to history. Many of the dairy herds around Thirsk have wound up – when I first practised there were around seventy within a ten-mile radius; nowadays there are about four in the same area – and the farm where Marcus used to work now has a pair of robots rather than a cowman. It's good for the cows and efficient but, of course, at the expense of a farm job. Marcus had made a successful, non-farming job for himself and judging by the width of the smile on his face, was enjoying it. ("I still miss me cows, though," he would always admit.)

"I hope your bottle of wine goes down better than the whisky in the cow, Marcus," I said by way of goodbye.

"Aye, so do I!"

Boston, Lincs.

Boston, Lincolnshire is not on everyone's list of weekend destinations, but I've been there a few times lately. The flat and foggy fenland has a long, straight watercourse called the River Haven. It's not an apt name, having the appearance of a huge, glorified drainage ditch. However, a five-kilometre reach, straight but for a single twenty-five-degree bend halfway along, makes this the perfect place for British Rowing to conduct its time trials for squad selection. Both my sons, Jack and Archie, have been racing there bidding for a place in the next round of selection for the GB team. Offering support and transporting boats has meant some very early mornings as well as logistical headaches in recent weekends.

Boston first came to my attention when I was at vet school. Michael, a good friend on the veterinary course, lived there and he loved the area, evangelising about his hometown at almost every opportunity. He was a funny and affable guy and became a popular vet, although at university he had more passion for and commitment to the local pub than the lecture theatre. Amusingly, during one of his final exams, the external examiner asked him if he had a job lined up after graduation.

"Yes, I'm going to work in Boston," Michael replied. The eyes of the high-powered examiner lit up immediately.

"Ah, Boston, Massachusetts. It's a fine university with an excellent veterinary department. I know the professor very well. Give him my regards." Michael was already heading for an easy pass. But his deadpan reply was not quite what the examiner was expecting,

"No, Boston Lincolnshire."

I think Mike still works in Boston. I should have looked him up whilst on my recent Boston sojourns, but watching rowing races is surprisingly time-consuming. Walking along the dead-straight river and waiting for scullers to pass, I checked a few Boston facts on my phone using Google and Wikipedia. It turned out there weren't many. Boston's most recent claim to fame was that the town achieved the highest percentage (75%) of votes in favour of Brexit in the 2016 referendum. This was ironic, because the few Boston facts I *could* find revealed its history to be intrinsically connected with Saxons, Vikings, Romans and people from Brittany. From a cursory inspection of the town, it didn't seem that Brexit had worked out terribly well for the locals. A field full of rotting, unharvested cabbages next to the river told its own story as strongly as the decomposing aroma it gave off. I'm guessing nobody was around to pick the produce.

But I'm no expert on cabbage farming, so back to the action on the water. During the first weekend, son number one, Jack, did very well indeed. He was the youngest rower there, and also the smallest. The first guy to row past me, as I watched and waited, was the world record holder and most of the next ten had rowed in the Olympics. A result of 28th overall and third amongst the under 21s was exceptional and augurs well for the next stage.

The next weekend, son number two, Archie, was in action, also young in his category but aiming to impress for selection for the under-19 team. Taller, leaner, more angular but less experienced, his confidence was rightly high, and he was excited. In his favour, and compared to his older brother, none of his competitors held world records and nobody had competed in the Olympics. At least, not yet.

The weekend was equally successful. Archie raced over two days and was comfortably within the top ten on both, confirming progress to the next stage: squad training. The diary at home, already pretty jam-packed, has suddenly been filled with pencilled-in dates for training camps, more trials and races across Europe. I'll keep you posted…

Henges

Boris excitedly munched on the succulent leaves of the two newly planted shrubs. To save the day, or at least to save the plants, Anne hastily constructed two, circular rabbit-proof fences.

"That'll teach you, Boris."

Later that day, we came across another rabbit-proof fence, this one much larger. We went to visit the amazing Neolithic henges at Thornborough, the custody of which has recently passed to Historic England to safeguard their future. The rabbit-proof fences were to prevent rabbits burrowing into the henges – another challenge these structures have faced over the years. Apparently, wild rabbits find them a superb home and simple to excavate for burrows. But the original purpose of the henges remains obscure.

I've been aware of these structures ever since I came to work in Thirsk in 1996. However, since they were on private land, until now it has been almost impossible to experience their history and majesty. A cold Sunday afternoon, with a pale sun approaching the horizon and stinging rain spitting in a north wind, provided a perfect opportunity to explore. Standing on the edge of the southernmost henge, with views to the east of Sutton Bank reflecting amber in the sunshine and with menacing clouds gathering over the Dales to the west, it was easy to sense the history of this place over the past six millennia. Thousands of others must have done the same as me. Most of them without the benefit of a warm fleece jacket, thick down coat and woolly hat. Although, I suppose, even Neolithics would have been dressed for the weather, probably with *literally* a fleece! Different to us today, but maybe, in some ways –worries, anxieties, hopes and dreams – very similar.

The three circular henges are arranged on the elevated plateau between the Ure and the Swale in an almost straight line. The northern-most is covered in trees and we didn't visit that one, but the central and southern circles are easy to see. The banks are somewhat subsided now (pesky rabbits again, as well as pesky other things) but, apparently, they were once four or five metres high, offering a grandstand view of whatever was going on in the central area. Also, investigations suggest that they were covered in gypsum, mined from pits nearby, so they would have had striking light and shiny surfaces. I imagined they reflected the evening sun in just the same way as the Sutton Bank escarpment was doing just now.

It was easy to imagine this impressive arena was a central venue for Neolithic man (and woman) in Northern England. There is speculation that the equally impressive and obscure and equally Neolithic Devil's Arrows, standing stones twenty miles to the south, just outside Boroughbridge, may have acted as an early signpost to these huge henges, pointing the way for visitors from the south 4,500 years before Christ.

Thornborough's big (very big) brother, Stonehenge, is aligned with the rising sun in midsummer and the setting sun in midwinter. Yorkshire's similar circles also have their southern entrances lined up with sunrise at the winter solstice. It's all fascinating. How and why our ancient ancestors created these amazing structures are unanswerable questions. Anne and my theory was that they were the sight of an ancient sporting event or a massive party. Competitors from all over Neolithic Britain (though it wasn't called that back then, of course), might have travelled to run around the circular track, then onto the next? Two and a half thousand years before the Greeks. That these henges still exist in 2023 and we can stand in the same circular places and wonder and try to empathise is bewildering. And it's most definitely worth a visit. Like our newly planted shrubs, I just hope the rabbits don't demolish them!

Crufts

Partly because there wasn't much on telly and partly because it's incumbent on a vet to remain up to date with modern trends, we watched some of the action at Crufts last weekend. I have to say, it's not my usual cup of tea, but Anne insists it is essential viewing. The bits I saw reminded me a bit of Eurovision, with a strong emphasis on performance and visual impact. I'd been invited to attend this annual dog festival in person on a few occasions, but never managed to make it. So, once again, I watched from the sofa.

In the early rounds, our eyes were drawn towards a dog in the working category. This fluffy character – which looked very much like a sturdy cockapoo, but was in fact a Lagotto Romagnolo – stood out as a fine specimen. His coat was immaculate and his markings looked as if he was wearing a smart woollen tank top. The breed was not one that either of us had come across before. As Peter Purves explained, its role had evolved from hunting ducks in Italy, to finding truffles. This gentle pastime seemed to fit very nicely with the dog's jolly demeanour. We watched as besuited judges, dressed as smartly as any Harley Street consultant, lifted tails and palpated shoulders and jaws. Was this really a thorough assessment, I wondered? Nevertheless, he made it through to the next round and we switched over to continue with our harrowing trip to *Happy Valley*.

By Sunday evening, it was time for a recap of some of the best bits. Dancing dogs and athletic collies dashing over, round and under things provided some excitement and drama. I looked at Emmy asleep in her beanbag and wondered if she still had the potential to do the agility. Maybe next year? One thing was for certain, we both stood no chance in the dancing dog/owner competition. Soon, the drama of "Best in Show" was approaching. Owners and dogs paraded around the ring and it was hard to say whether the canine or the human was enjoying it most. A wolfhound with luxurious long and flowing hair covered the ground effortlessly. A standard poodle was next with different hair altogether. Peter Purves explained the haircut was functional – the bulbous fluff around the carpal joints was designed to keep the legs warm whilst swimming to collect ducks from cold lakes. And the shaved rear end allowed improved streamlining through the water. Apparently.

The little fluffy truffle-hunter was back, enjoying his second time in the ring. His tail continued to wag and Anne and I again agreed he should win. With one more circumnavigation of the ring for each dog, the tension was rising. Peter announced that the chief judge had made his decision and he wandered over to a table to sign some important documents before the final announcement. This was the perfect time to build jeopardy and cut to a commercial break, which was littered with adverts for allegedly super-tasty and uber-healthy dog foods, which lived in the fridge next to the yoghurts. We could hardly wait until the coverage resumed.

The judge had made his judgement. First, he strode purposefully to an Old English sheepdog. It was a fine specimen and deserving of reserve champion. As tension reached a crescendo, the judge marched over to the Lagotto, whose name was Orca, and shook hands with his delighted (and rather surprised) owner. Cameras snapped as the champion stood on a podium next to a huge trophy, an emerald green rosette and an enormous bottle of champagne. Whether Orca was aware of his monumental achievement was not clear. One thing was for sure: his tail had not stopped wagging all week. That, alone, deserved the prize.

Opening Libraries

By coincidence, I've been asked to open the newly revamped and restocked libraries of two primary schools recently. Until last Monday, the only things that I had officially opened were a Christmas tree shop on the outskirts of Easingwold and a bike shop in Thirsk. School libraries are in a totally different league because it's a positive contribution to the next generation. I was delighted to help. There was sure to be a ribbon to cut and possibly even a plaque! At our local swimming pool, there is a plaque commemorating its opening, some years ago, by William Hague, then MP for Richmond. I wondered if a similar one (or two) had been hewn with my name. There hadn't been one at the Christmas tree emporium or the bicycle shop, so I didn't get my hopes up.

The first school was in Leeds. In advance, I tried to prepare but I really hoped nobody would expect a reading from my latest book. I'm told this is what authors do as a matter of routine when attending literary events or opening libraries, but it never sits comfortably with me. When I was at school, I hated reading out loud from books in class. Nowadays, especially when the text has been written by me, it's not quite so bad, but I still don't like it and I'm not very good at it. I tried to explain this to a friend, who happens to be a performance poet, as she assured me that it was essential to read out an appropriate passage.

"Yes, but it just feels a bit 'showy-offy'," I pleaded, but she wasn't convinced.

I rushed out of the practice during my lunch break. With just a couple of hours before I had to be back for afternoon surgery, I'd have to be succinct. The opening went to plan and the children seemed thrilled to have a real-life vet and author sitting on the sofa of their new library. I snipped the ribbon, was interviewed by two reporters from the school magazine and signed some books. It was every bit as straightforward as the Christmas trees and bikes. And there was no plaque, which pleased me – it was much better to channel all available funds into actual books.

Buoyed by the simplicity of this task, I felt more relaxed about my next library-opening event, which was in the middle of the North York Moors. In advance, I'd spoken to the head teacher over the phone.

"Most of the children at the school are from farming families and it can be challenging to find books that capture their interest," she explained. "But two of our pupils have taken your book home and read it from cover to cover. That's never happened before. We'd love it if you could come and visit."

I'd been thinking about writing books for a younger audience for a while. I knew it would be difficult, but the challenge was appealing. *Adventures of a Yorkshire Vet: Lambing Time and Other Tales* was certainly the hardest book I've written. But I'd seen the huge impact *The Yorkshire Vet* has had (and continues to have) on its fans, many of whom are young people. Some have been inspired to follow a career working with animals as a result. I had an email a couple of months ago from a lady whose daughter, Emily, had watched our programme on Channel 5, read my books, then applied to vet school. She'd just graduated as a veterinary surgeon. The genuine gratitude in the email from Emily's mum was touching. I don't know how many 8- to 11-year-olds (the book's target audience) will follow in my or Emily's veterinary footsteps having read my collection of winter animal stories. But for me it's been worth it, if Yorkshire has just two more young bibliophiles.

Libraries (2)

Gillamoor School was the venue for my second library opening. Perched in a remote spot near the edge of a windswept moor, I sensed that the kids would probably have a slightly different set of experiences to the Leeds pupils from my previous library trip. When I arrived, they were sitting politely, ready and eagerly waiting in the small hall. The hall doubled up as a classroom as well as the dining room.

"The space is quite limited here, but we make the most of what we have," explained the head teacher. "We are a small school and it's a small community. But we do our best."

Before any ribbon cutting was done, we had a detailed discussion and question-asking session. Immediately, hands shot up. Talking to school kids is always great, because their enormous enthusiasm is so infectious. One young lad, Emerson, talked about the small but expanding flock of sheep he owned – his first lambing time was approaching. Another explained his love of tractors, his capabilities around repairing them and his favourite model. Someone else explained about the family's farm shop and all the vegetables they produce and sell. Another talked about showing pigeons – including at the Yorkshire Show. Apparently, it's standard practice to shampoo them with washing-up liquid!

The ceremonial opening was simple, and it was great to experience another wonderfully stocked library. Sensing the possible demand for animal books, I left a copy of my children's book to add to the shelves. I'd been invited to stay for lunch and sit with some of the kids so we could talk a little bit more. I queued up and was shown where to stand and where to collect my plate. Surrounded by small people and about to sit on a tiny chair, I felt like a giant. Primary school teachers must feel like giants all the time. The sausages and mash looked delicious and came with three types of vegetables. The kids at Gillamoor were well fed as well as well read! Emerson was clearly excited about his imminent lambing time and voiced some of his concerns. He didn't have much experience or knowledge so far. As I finished my yoghurt, I found myself volunteering to help. I hoped he'd take me up on the offer, because I think giving him some help and guidance would be great. Another boy told me more about his family's suckler herd and his sheep. Lambing and calving would be starting before long, but there was no lack of experience on his farm. Farming was in his blood.

I helped tidy away the plates and did a few photos, but there was only so long I could linger in the school.

"Thank you for inviting me and I'm really sorry I've ruined your day of proper teaching!"

"Absolutely not – this is what education is all about!" exclaimed the head. "The kids will remember today for a long time!"

As I left Gillamoor's lovely little school, I felt very pleased to have visited. It had been a great and enlightening experience. I reflected on the next generation of farmers and animal lovers, possibly even one or two veterinary surgeons. There had been some wonderful conversations and discussions. I'd enjoyed my lunch, the opening of the library and meeting the staff too. But my favourite moment, and a recollection that I hope will stay with me for ever was during our question-and-answer session. A boy on the front row had been patiently sitting with his hand raised. When I signalled to him to ask his question he simply said,

"Last night I had a dream about a sausage."

The head teacher smiled, as we all did in response to such a funny thing, before quietly adding, "Welcome to our world."

Lambing Time

This week, I had a call during evening surgery. On old friend, a farmer, was having trouble with one of his shearlings. She'd started lambing and seemed to be in difficulty. Could I come and help?

We have a flexible and informal relationship to veterinary care on his farm. It's one where everyone is happy. Rodney calls me if he has a problem. If I'm free and available, I go over to help. If not, then his regular vet comes to assist. This evening, although I was just finishing evening surgery after a busy day, I pledged my assistance.

"I'll be able to set off in about twenty minutes, if that's OK?" I said. It was. Soon, I was en route to my first lambing of the season.

I was soon rolling up my sleeves, filling my bucket with water (cold) and antiseptic solution and grabbing a bottle of lubricant. I have known Rodney for about eight years and treated many of his animals. Sheep which have needed lambing or prolapses replaced, goats who needed their horn buds removing – not a job that many vets relish – and, of course, some veterinary care for his beloved Border collies. Millie, many years ago, needed a cancerous tumour on her lower jaw to be surgically removed. The local vet had shied away from tackling the task, but it went very well. Millie lived until an old age. The matriarch of the farm and leader of the pack, she continued enthusiastically helping with the sheep until well beyond her sixteenth birthday. Flynn, an exuberant but haphazard youngster, suffered a nasty fracture to his humerus after crashing into a stationary tractor provided me with another challenge. Happily, he is still well, very mobile and trying to help gather up sheep.

But this evening was all about the sheep. Rodney caught the shearling, which was standing alone in the corner of the pen, with ease. He explained to me that all the sheep knew him well, and that he spoke to them all and he listened to them in turn. There was a strong bond between this amazing farmer and his flock. I really hoped I'd be able to cajole the lamb out. I prepared my hand and arm and readied myself for the initial inspection. It's always the moment of truth because there is a multitude of scenarios that can exist. Tonight, the lamb was presented in one of the worst positions – it was breech. This means the lamb is coming backside and tail first. It is backwards, with its hind legs flexed forwards so they are pointing towards the sheep's head. There is no way a lamb can be born this way, so careful manipulation is required to get the legs round and pointing out backwards.

Of course, I had a camera following my every move, eager to capture the exciting story for a future episode of *The Yorkshire Vet*. Commentating to camera has become second nature these days, and I did my best to describe what I could feel and what I was trying to do. As the moments went by, I'd managed to dilate the birth canal and then correct the position of first one, then the other leg. I was winning, but still the lamb needed to be delivered. It is a balance between allowing the birth canal to dilate naturally, while not being too slow and risking the suffocation of the lamb. There is a big risk of this with posterior presentations, especially if the umbilical cord is wrapped around a back leg.

But there were no such problems this evening, and the lamb was soon extracted. We cleared its airways and settled it on the straw in front of the new mum. My work was done, but the mum's evening – and Rodney's – was just beginning…

Opening the Fridge

Alison sounded fraught, her voice strained with worry and frustration.

"They've learnt how to open the fridge!"

I raised my eyebrows.

The dogs looked very pleased with themselves, with vigorously wagging tails and wide, salivating grins. None of them showed even the vaguest signs of illness – in fact, quite the opposite. Knowing that Labradors and setters enjoy a challenge, and also like food, it was easy to understand why they were so happy.

Alison went on to explain. Whilst she was out, the three dogs had managed to open the fridge.

"It was only last week that they opened the cupboard and ate all the birdseed. It's Carrie that's the instigator," she said.

After the success in the cupboard (which turned out not to have been so successful, because Carrie was very poorly), it was only a matter of time before they turned their attention to more ambitious heists. I had visions of the dogs standing on one another's shoulders, in a sort of canine pyramid. I'd once dealt with a flock of sheep who had broken into a stable block and, for some reason, eaten lumps of rat poison. A similar image came to mind back then, like a scene from a *Wallace and Gromit* film. Why do they do these things?

Some of the sheep didn't do very well after that nocturnal feast, as it was impossible to identify which had ingested the toxin and impractical to treat the whole flock with antidote.

Another patient, one I sadly had to put down a few months ago, was also adept at opening things he shouldn't. As I administered the final injection at home, in familiar and calm surroundings, we reminisced about the long and full life of the shaggy mongrel. I knew some of the stories from his life, but by no means all.

"And one day, he learnt how to open a jar of marmalade!" said his owner. "I got home and discovered he'd eaten the lot. His fuzzy face was totally sticky with orange bits everywhere. He was a sticky mess. But he was such a funny dog. I'm really gonna miss him."

Luckily, and somewhat miraculously, Alison's menagerie escaped without serious illness, although she confessed, "There was a bit of vomiting."

"So, what happened?" I asked.

"Well, I got home from work and the kitchen was a complete mess. The fridge door was open and empty packets were strewn everywhere."

"What have they devoured?" I asked, my mind starting to scroll through a list of the potentially poisonous foods that might have been swallowed. Chocolate puddings or cakes, or anything containing onions, for example, have very specific toxicities. But other things might simply cause an upset tummy or be an expensive mistake. It was important to know.

Alison reeled off the list, just like you might dictate a shopping list, or the weekly intake of a very hungry but very unhealthy caterpillar. There was one packet of butter, two cartons of margarine, three packets of cheese. But worse! The greedy hounds had eaten all the tomatoes!

Robyn, our witty nurse, quickly retorted, "If only they'd found the bread, they could have made some lovely sandwiches!"

But was it the time to be joking? we wondered. The gastroenterologist part of me fretted about the health of the dogs' pancreases. So much fatty food can play havoc with this delicate digesting organ. But the thrifty Yorkshireman in me went cold upon hearing that this now most expensive commodity had been snaffled.

"NOT THE TOMATOES!"

At least the cucumbers and peppers, safe in the salad compartment, had survived the attack! Performing some quick mental arithmetic, I said, "That must have cost you about £35!"

"Yes, but now I've got a child lock. It won't happen again."

Complicated Surgery

Is it the case that surgical procedures with a complicated name are more difficult than those with simple names? A "spay" sounds much more straightforward than an "ovariohysterectomy" but is the same procedure, while a "tie-back" sounds as simple as fastening a shoelace. Its proper name, "Unilateral Arytenoid Lateralisation" sounds much more technical, which it very much is.

The surgery in store for me this week certainly fell into the complicated category. A rostral mandibulectomy isn't for the fainthearted. For the owner, the patient or the surgeon. I had seen Ollie as a second opinion. I read the clinical notes and examined the painful, invasive tumour that was eating into the bone of his lower jaw. Just as important as the examination was the ensuing discussion with Ollie's owner. I explained the prognosis and the options for Ollie. The tumour was clearly aggressive and, without something drastic, the poor chap would certainly need to be put to sleep before long – a matter of weeks rather than months. Although he was quite old, Ollie's general health was good. I've never been a fan of avoiding surgery simply on the grounds of age. Human surgeons don't ignore the fractured hip of an old lady based on her age, so why should vets? The procedure with the complicated name would allow me to remove the cancerous bone, but also the front part of Ollie's jaw. I explained what would be involved and the post-operative implications, one of which was that his tongue would lol out of his mouth, certainly temporarily, if not permanently. There would be plenty of post-op analgesics and nerve blocks, like when we go to the dentist. The biggest challenge for Ollie would be to learn how to eat with a modified mouth. I related some examples of other surgeries I had done of this type: Milly, a farm dog who, into her mid-teens, could still round up sheep with her tongue hanging out; Alfie, the cocker spaniel, is just as old and totally recovered from the same surgery I performed many years ago. Since then, he's had an anal gland tumour removed and is now having a platelet deficiency treated. Despite a multitude of problems over his life, he continues to be happy.

"And modern dogs don't use their front teeth for eating food," I explained. "In antiquity, they were used for pulling at the hides of the prey they had caught. In the days when they had to hunt for their food. On a modern diet, the front part of the jaw is broadly redundant."

Ollie's owner went away to consider the best course of action, and quickly decided to go ahead. On the morning of the op, I got to work early so I could focus and have a clear head. We talked through the procedure again and everyone was happy. Apart, that is, from our new nurse, who was still in her first week. Although Kelly had years of experience, I hadn't operated with her before. As I inserted the battery to the oscillating saw, there was a tense excitement in theatre. Inspecting the X-rays and the abnormal bone of Ollie's jaw, I judged where to make the first cut. Running down the middle of the mandible is a major artery, amusingly called the *mental artery* and, surrounded by bone, it is hard to ligate. Blood can spurt in a continuous and disconcerting way, before the diathermy finally does its thing. Kelly remained impressively calm throughout and, before too long, Ollie's tumour was off and I set about reconstructing the area where there had once been bone.

A few days later, he was back for a check-up.

"It's amazing!" exclaimed his owner. "He's much more comfortable than before the operation, and look," she showed me a video on her phone, "he can already eat all by himself!"

Ferret Castration; Ferret Vasectomy

Last Monday I had two ferrets on my ops list. For some vets, this might be cause for consternation. Ferrets are quirky creatures. Some people love them, others don't. Yes, they are smelly and occasionally unpredictable and, as Richard Whiteley testified back in the 1970s, they have very sharp teeth. When they find their target – a rabbit or a TV presenter – they cling on tenaciously. But I am a ferret fan. I've loved them since I was small boy. On my first day at secondary school, when I was eleven, the task during English was to go to the library and "find a book". Of course, it was an exercise to teach new pupils how to make use of the library. In the days before Google, it was where we got our information. My classmates searched for books about football, cricket or academic topics, but I had the librarian flummoxed – the school did not have a single book on the topic of "Ferrets and Ferreting". I was disappointed and my first day at big school was not off to an illustrious start.

In the present day, my knowledge of these curious creatures has expanded and doesn't seem to have been hindered by the shortage of literature available to me as a boy. Both the ferrets required surgery on their nether regions, but different procedures with markedly different outcomes. The first, a rescue ferret called Brian was simple enough. He needed to be castrated. This is an excellent way to reduce the masculine impulses, allow the male to cohabit happily with other males without fighting and with females without mating. And, with hormones removed, the smell subsides considerably.

For Bruce, contestant number two, the testicular surgery was very different. In fact, it was vastly different (a joke I made almost continuously, much to the annoyance of everyone within earshot). Bruce was in for a vasectomy.

"Why would a ferret need a vasectomy?" I hear you ask. The answer lies in the peculiar reproductive cycle of the female of the species. Female ferrets, called jills, are *induced ovulators*. This means they only ovulate after they have been mated. It's a great way to increase the chances of becoming pregnant and, in ferret circles at least, an evolutionary advantage. The downside for the jill is that the persistent state of oestrus leads to prolonged periods of high oestrogen. Not only can this be irksome, but it's downright dangerous. High oestrogen can suppress the bone marrow, leading to life-threatening anaemia. There are several ways to reduce this risk, but one tried, tested and foolproof way is to let them be mated. If the male is vasectomised, the jill comes out of season, her bone marrow is spared and she doesn't become pregnant. This was today's fiddly job. It was a job for an extra powerful pair of glasses because the vas deferens, which needed to be identified, ligated and transected, is about 1 mm wide. The vas deferens is the pale pink tube which takes sperm from the testicle to the penis, and thence to the female. Finding the tube – one coming from each testicle – was as difficult as it sounds. To make matters worse, each time the area was palpated and manipulated in an effort to identify the correct part of anatomy, another wave of pungent ferret smell would flood through theatre like a tsunami. It's very difficult to describe the nature, extent and potency of male ferret pheromone. It makes the eyes sting and forces swear words out of the mouth, although not for long, because if you leave your mouth open for more than a split second, the smell turns into a taste. Forty years ago, had I managed to find that book, I bet it wouldn't have mentioned this in my book review!

Naughty Gus

Gus is a one-year-old Spaniel. He is lovely but a very naughty boy. His first misdemeanour was a couple of months ago when he chewed up and swallowed a collar with a transponder. The main problem was nobody knew whether the culprit was Gus or one of his friends – Orla the Labrador and Nixxi the Spaniel. Each dog looked similarly guilty, so there was nothing for it but to make them all sick. This is not something to be done lightly. Vets spend much time *stopping* dogs from being sick. To deliberately inject an emetic to induce vomiting seems very mean. However, the balance between benefit and harm needs to be weighed up. The possibility of a chewed-up transponder obstructing the bowel and necessitating surgery, in this case, outweighed the unpleasantness of being made sick. To digress briefly, at last someone has worked out that the toxic dose of raisins or grapes is dose dependent, rather than just "any". This means that your dog's out-of-hours emergency may not be an emergency if we can estimate the number of raisins swallowed in relation to the dog's weight. Hopefully, many dogs can be spared the trauma of vet-induced-vomiting.

But back to Gus. Thankfully, every single chewed-up bit of collar came up, but only out of Gus's stomach. Naughty Gus. Poor Orla and Nixxi looked very forlorn having brought up their collar-free breakfasts.

A few weeks later, Orla was back. Her owner was concerned about the recent increase in size. "Could she have a growth internally?"

This was a possibility, but very unlikely in an eight-month-old Labrador. There was another, more likely, diagnosis. "Is there any chance Orla could be pregnant?" Vigorous shaking of the head followed, but the ultrasound scan revealed the very opposite. Two weeks later, nine very cute, but very unplanned Labrador-cross-Spaniel puppies entered the world.

"That bloody Gus!"

As the pups' eyes opened and as they grew and prospered under the care of Orla the teenage mum, Gus still had ambitions. The next week, the family were back on the phone. He'd been at it again; this time, caught in the act with Nixxi.

"Bloody Gus has been at it again. This time with Nixxi! I found them together on the sofa."

Luckily, this time we were in a better position to solve the problem before it became one (or several). The canine equivalent of the morning after pill is two injections, administered on consecutive days. This would ensure the household was not overrun with another cute but unexpected litter of pups.

At this point, Gus's owner was considering pitching a tent on the grass outside our practice because she was spending so much time at our clinic. But we had another, much more permanent plan to solve at least one of Gus's issues. Gus was duly booked in for castration. "I was planning to use him for breeding and having a litter at some point. He's so lovely, but I've had enough. I just can't cope with any more."

Gus appeared one morning at the surgery as arranged and we prepared him for surgery. As the premedication was taking effect, his one and only litter, carried in a large laundry basket, was receiving their first vaccinations. This was the fifth visit in not very long. The bill was growing, but at least an end was in sight. By the afternoon, Gus's testicles were disconnected from the rest of him and at least one of the problems had been solved.

The final visit, ten days later, Gus returned, wagging his tail cheerfully as usual, for us to check his healing. Anne looked into his appealing eyes. "Yes, and butter still wouldn't melt, would it, Gus?"

Race Mode

Last week, I was back in race mode. I had not been in this competitive frame of mind since last August when my eldest son, Jack, and I completed the Swiss Epic five-day mountain bike race. Its name was apt. This time the race was just one day. The Top of the Rock Race started from the top of Sutton Bank rather than a village high in the Swiss Alps, although the distance, height gain, beauty and challenge were very similar. Despite age catching up with me – if not overtaking me quite yet I felt – I was up for the challenge.

I'd entered on a whim. It was local and I reckoned I knew the tracks and trails like the back of my hand. It was described as a "Gravel Bike Ride" but that did not put me off. I do not own a gravel bike, nor have I ever been tempted. For me, dropped handlebars are for riding on the road. If you venture off road and into muddier, steeper, rockier and bumpier places, you need a different bike altogether. The blurb suggested that the long course – 53 miles, with nearly 2,000 metres of ascent – was also suitable for people riding mountain bikes. I was interested to see if these new-fangled gravel bike things could really cope. I oiled my mountain bike, pumped up the knobbly tyres and greased my dropper post.

I was fit and confident. If the entry list was short, I even fancied my chances of winning. Over many years of competition, I should have learnt by now that this outcome is extremely unlikely. Always optimistic, when it comes to claiming a prize, I usually end up disappointed. But this was my patch. Surely that would carry an advantage?

I'd checked the route online. I recognised the course. Of course, it would all be signposted with arrows stuck to trees and bushes, and there would be a map too.

At registration, early on Sunday morning, I was handed said map and a timing chip. "Is it all signposted?" I asked an official. "Yes.

Have you downloaded the GPX file of the route? It's all very clear on that." I made an excuse about the link not having worked. In reality, I am not technically very savvy and I don't really know what a GPX file is, nor how I could get it onto my Garmin bike computer. If I could have, I think it would have provided me with accurate instructions. But with a waterproof map in my pocket and lots of local knowledge, I thought I'd be fine.

I set off at high speed. After the first couple of miles, I was cruising. I'd overtaken about six people, mostly struggling on gravel bikes, through mud and on a gentle descent. I whizzed along with skill and confidence with my wide, grippy tyres and subtle suspension. It was going very well. Within the first hour, I was already predicting a record finishing time. I flew down and through a farm where I once had calved heifers, treated calf pneumonia cases and even helped with the clinical trials of a new drug.

But then, disaster struck. Near Rievaulx, I went the wrong way. Two crucial signs had been removed overnight by rascals. I followed my instinct but wasted half an hour heading in the wrong direction. I checked the map, but to no avail. The writing and detail was too tiny and I had not thought to bring my reading glasses. The minute detail of the route on the small trails around the upper reaches of the river Rye was simply impossible to see, let alone read. It seemed that I had indeed been overtaken by age, as well as a few other cyclists. I wasn't going to win.

Catching Up

From the moment I whizzed at full pelt in the wrong direction, I was playing catch-up. Regardless of the type of bike I was on and its capability over different terrain, my ambitions of being the fastest rider had all but gone. Despite my utter inability to see the tiny details on my map, I knew approximately where I should be and where the first checkpoint was. Overlooking the quaint village of Hawnby, I'd passed the place many times, both on two wheels and in the course of my veterinary duties. Once, I'd performed a challenging caesarean on a wild heifer in a freezing and draughty barn just a hundred yards from the checkpoint. Fortunately, I had found a track that put me back on track. On a fast descent, I came across an unfortunate guy on his gravel bike. Or, more accurately, off his gravel bike. On the bumpy track, without the benefit of suspension, his phone had bounced out of his pocket and was lost in the mud.

"Can you phone me up?" he pleaded. "If the phone rings, I might hear it."

I was happy to help, but we couldn't hear any ringing. More precious minutes passed, driving another nail into the coffin for my chances of winning this race.

I sped along more muddy tracks, increasingly convinced that my mountain bike was superior to the gravel bike alternative. So far, they appeared totally incapable of progressing downhill with any degree of competency, and on a climb up Hasty Bank near Pockley, gravel riders were pushing UP hill as well. Thin tyres lacked grip and apparently the gears weren't right either. The tyres on my bike were great and so were the gears. I was fine.

Before long, I found myself on the bleak Pockley Moor. At a gate, I caught up with two more mountain bikers. We chatted for a while, about the fantastic course and the wonderful places we were enjoying this chilly Sunday and about the benefits and deficiencies of the two types of vélo on show.

"Hey, are you The Yorkshire Vet?" one of them asked in a thick Leeds accent. In the middle of a muddy moor, with only half the distance completed, it seemed irrelevant to me. I nodded.

"That's med me day," he replied with a grin.

Where the track across Pockley Moor met a road, there was a feed station. These places provide racers with more water, biscuits, sweets, and hope. There were more people too. A mate who works in a local bike shop happened to be out on a ride. He'd stopped to have a chat and grab some free sweets. Another old face grinned from under a wide pair of sunglasses.

"Julian, how's it going? We met last year on a Thursday evening bike ride. You came with Ben." I remembered the ride. Everyone there (except me) was of Olympic ability and, I'm sure, could have held Tom Pidcock's wheel for at least a few metres. This was Guy, with his mate Graham, two skilled, fit and talented riders. I was delighted to have met them and we rode together for the final twenty miles, opening gates for one another and sharing the lead. Amusingly, Guy said "Thanks, love" to anyone who held open a gate for him, which was nice.

The final stretches, desperately clinging to Guy's wheel, were speedy (thanks, love) despite mounting fatigue. The printout at the finish confirmed that at least four people were faster than me, two of whom were Guy and Graham. Reflecting on a great day, but a mildly disappointing final position, I realised I needed to add one more item to my kit list, to help me see the map: my reading glasses.

Death by Mince Pie

Maggie was in with her elderly owners, Mr and Mrs C, for another appointment. The usually effervescent cocker spaniel had been suffering from a vague and slightly obscure malaise. Blood tests had not revealed much, but her high temperature and subdued demeanour had improved after a course of antibiotics.

Today, Maggie was back to normal, the thermometer read a happy and healthy 38.5 degrees. Bang on normal. I still could not find any anomalies, despite a thorough clinical examination. This is always irksome, because logic would suggest that it should be simple to find the cause of pyrexia (high temperature).

"She's feeling much better," explained Mrs C, "but I have noticed one thing since last time we were here. Maggie has been behaving oddly; doing strange things. She's been acting as if she has dementia." That gave me a clue as to the actual diagnosis, something that's notoriously difficult to detect, even with the benefits of modern techniques.

"I think she may have had a kidney infection," I declared with some confidence. "It's quite common in dogs, hard to confirm but often causes a high temperature. And, a bit like in old people, it can cause confusion." This empirical fact is not (to my knowledge) written down in any veterinary textbook, but it is something I have noticed over the years. Why it happens, nobody knows. Or, at least, I don't know.

"That would make sense," concurred Mr C, before adding, "The same thing happened to my step mother-in-law, several years ago."

I nodded and smiled, awaiting the story, which was sure to follow. I've known Maggie's owners for many years, and they are a double act, always grateful for the treatment of their dogs and usually equipped with a funny anecdote.

"She seemed to think drinking whisky was the answer. But it didn't really help. The more she drank, the harder it was for her to get out of bed to go for a wee, which only made the problem worse. Eventually, in hospital, they worked it out and got her sorted. Then she stopped being so confused."

I agreed. It sounded similar to Maggie's condition, although fortunately no whisky was involved.

"She was always causing problems," Mr C explained. "She died during a Christmas party we had several years ago in Scotland. She choked on a mince pie." This surely would surpass all previous anecdotes.

"I was sitting next to her and I didn't even notice," he explained, loudly and, surprisingly, with some amusement. "Her head just lolled forward, but I thought she had fallen asleep like usual."

More details about the mince pie incident followed. "Yes, it got stuck but it was too far in to get at. Luckily, one of the family was a nurse, and she performed the Heimlich manoeuvre. But it was to no avail. We couldn't get it out. If only we had realised she didn't have her false teeth in that day. It turned out she hadn't been able to chew her beef properly either. We'll never know if that contributed, but it was the mince pie that was the final straw. Well, the final pie I suppose."

"Yes," continued Mrs C, "it was like an episode of an Agatha Christie novel with a dead person lying on the floor of the dining room. We'll never forget that Christmas."

By now, despite the sad end to their step mother-in-law, but buoyed by the happier news of Maggie's recovery, I couldn't stop laughing at the scene they had painted. Maggie was signed off. I didn't need to see her again, although secretly I hoped she would be back before too long, because, animal ailment or not, I really, really enjoyed it when the family came to see me.

Jess and the Magic Spell

Jess always makes me smile. The springer spaniel has been an accident-prone extrovert from a very young age. The series of mild calamities could have graced pages of a veterinary emergency textbook. Some of her early ailments included conjunctivitis from bounding headlong into bracken, a sore nose after she shoved it into a hole and found a hedgehog at the bottom and a bout of terrible diarrhoea from eating a complete, decomposing rabbit carcass.

As an adolescent, Jess suffered numerous injuries to her tail. It wagged so much, and she didn't consider the consequences of bush jumping. "This dog is a nightmare!" her owner would declare with exasperation each time a trauma necessitated a visit to the vet. Eventually, the tail needed to be amputated, which went smoothly enough. Bandages were required, which had to be changed every three days. The first, I applied, but the job was simple enough and Jess's owner was extremely capable. But after the third new bandage, Jess and her owner were back again with another problem: Jess was straining to pass faeces. Could it be colitis? Or possibly constipation? Jess's mum relayed the story:

"Well, Julian. I thought I'd got quite good at re-bandaging the tail – the first one I tried fell off, but the second was OK and the third, well, I thought, 'This is a beauty, it's never going to come off.' I'd put on extra tape and it was great. Anyway, later that evening, as I took her out for a final walk I noticed that she was straining a bit. I thought to myself, 'Oh no! Not a bout of colitis. That's the last thing we need, what with a tail bandage and everything.' She came back into the house and then I thought, 'What's that strange smell?' and then I realized, I'd bandaged the tail, but also her BUM! I was mortified! She was trying to go to the toilet but couldn't because my bandage had gone all the way round her bottom! I felt awful and I cut it off immediately. I hope there's no lasting damage!"

Back then, Jess's temporarily obstructed bowels made a full

recovery and so did her tail. But the sight of a lame spaniel in the waiting room made me more worried than any badly placed bandage could. There is a multitude of reasons why a spaniel could be holding its front leg off the ground, and the worst is something called a condylar fracture.

When examining for lameness, I always start at the bottom of the limb and work my way upwards. First, feeling and bending each toe, then feeling between each pad. Next, I squeeze each pad in turn. Then, I move up to the carpus (our wrist), bend it and check for swellings or effusions. After a quick check of the middle bit (the antebrachium) to rule out a fracture, bone tumour or injury, I get busy with the elbow. Flexing and extending and pronating. Luckily, there was absolutely no pain or discomfort here. I was sure there was no nasty fracture. Finally, it's the shoulder. Harder to assess, the shoulder can be a subtle joint. It's a nice one to examine and requires gentle but firm palpation. I always explore the front part, called the bicipital groove, with my thumb.

But, after all her previous problems, Jess was lucky this time: one of her pads was sore. I could see a small hole and squeezed. With typical flamboyance, a six-millimetre blackthorn shot out of the hole, flew through the air and landed about three feet away, on the floor. Painful, for sure, but after a thorough examination it was a simple fix than any of her previous problems. It wasn't magic, but it was a spell.

Melancholy; Vultures

In an otherwise pleasant mid-summer, the persistent presence of low, light grey cloud seemed melancholy, stifling the emotions along with any movement of the leaves on the trees. It was chillier than expected too, making me wish I had put on an extra layer for the early morning dog walk. For a vet, melancholy moments are not uncommon. In the olden days, this was blamed on a disease called *Brucellosis*, which caused problems for cows, farmers and vets.

The ups and downs of clinical life are perennial. Cases don't always go to plan, especially in animals where bed rest or strict post-surgery rehabilitation regimes cannot be as easily enforced as they would in a cooperative human being. Dogs can lick their wounds, causing neatly placed sutures to become infected and sore, or chase after next door's cat when they should be resting; and they often do their best to avoid swallowing their medicine. Sometimes, it's hard to make a proper diagnosis, because of a host of practical limitations; but we must do the best we can, using our bank of experience and the support of colleagues. The cocker spaniel this afternoon, with a bleeding nose, a bleeding wart and bleeding gums was an example. I'd need a blood test to confirm a diagnosis of Immune Mediated Thrombocytopaenia, but I was confident I'd got it right and a traumatised and tearful owner left relieved that the diagnosis was prompt and the condition treatable.

Charlie, the thirteen-year-old golden retriever came in yesterday. I removed an aggressive anal gland tumour six months ago. At the time, it was touch and go whether we should undertake the surgery. Had the mass been much bigger, it would have been impossible to remove. So, it really was Charlie's last chance. But, he is doing remarkably well. The tumour has not reappeared and his visit to the practice was for a different, much milder condition. And Amore, who has an invasive and inoperable tumour, was in earlier this week. Miraculously, the metronomic chemotherapy regime has shrunk the mass, so it is almost impossible to detect. And her tail, like Charlie's, still wags. Two utterly positive outcomes, both against the odds. Most cases we see are not as dramatic as these and improve, get better, resolve, with simple treatment. But it only takes one or two cases that don't follow the expected course to batter your clinical confidence. I should have developed thicker skin by now. And I should have learnt that most things work out OK in the end, because or in spite of our intervention. But remembering that is sometimes easier said than done. I've been fortunate to have had innumerable occasions in which my confidence has been buoyed over the last few years. Confidence is something everyone needs to nurture, from the newly qualified veterinary nurse to the established doyen. Without it, everything is hard.

As I pondered whether it was time to hand over the reins to the next generation, with more energy and a modern perspective, a moment of levity improved my day: the work WhatsApp chat pinged into life. One of our new vets asked a question: "What's the ops list like on Monday? I have a vulture coming in for X-rays and blood tests." There was a flurry of different emojis as everyone responded and I couldn't help but laugh and added a reply: "The vultures are circling…" Given my mood, it seemed apt.

My week was improving, as the cloud lifted, the prospect of an evening on my bike became more real and the prognosis of my irksome cases improved. But the words of Clive James, as ever, crept into my head: "The melancholy will always come." The big question was whether the vultures would get here first.

Vultures

As it turned out, the vultures did arrive first. At least one of them did. Contrary to my imagination, it wasn't surveying the scene from overhead in ever decreasing circles. Rather he was transported in a big box, with secure fastenings and a wire door. Fluffy puppies turned their heads in surprise when they caught a glimpse of the contents of the box. So did most of the humans.

In recent years, I've witnessed some interesting inter-species interactions in the waiting room. One of the funniest was when two fully grown alpacas walked in, both on leads and head collars, as one needed a general anaesthetic to remove an internal testicle. The second came along for moral support, a metaphorical hand to hold. Or hoof, I suppose. Needless to say, there was more consternation in the waiting room that day.

Vultures have historically had a bad reputation, sitting hunched on bare branches or circling above weary desert travellers and awaiting their death. In times of antiquity, Aristotle and Pliny thought these birds signified bad luck and in ancient Egypt their association with gods (specifically Isis) caused people to dread them. Their habit of scavenging on the dead and their unnerving knack of arriving at the site of a carcass did nothing to help. However, their habit of *not* preying on or eating live animals confers vultures a sacred status in Tibet, where they are considered the protector and cleaner-up of the highest plateau in the world.

So, I didn't really know what to expect when the African white-backed vulture emerged from the box. He had come to Thirsk as part of a captive breeding project. They are critically endangered and teetering on the edge of extinction, as a result of human persecution. African poachers don't like them because their appearance alerts rangers to the presence of a recent kill. As a result, these horrible people try to poison the harmless birds. As if killing innocent rhinos or lions isn't egregious enough. We all really hoped that he would pass his health screening and be able to swell the numbers of his species once he met his mate.

His handlers, from Thirsk Birds of Prey Centre, introduced him as Vinnie. As the anaesthetic gas did its thing to send Vinnie to sleep and keep him still for the important X-rays to check his legs and to allow the blood sample to be collected, we could only watch in awe at this majestic bird. Far from being a menacing tyrant, delighting in death, Vinnie was a remarkable creature. His head and neck were devoid of proper feathers. Instead, this part of his body was covered in fluffy down, just like a baby bird, which made him look cute and appealing.

I'm not an expert in birds or exotic animals in general, so I asked questions to the knowledgeable owners with impunity. "Is that so his head doesn't get sticky with dried-up blood when he is chewing on carcasses?" I said. There was an enthusiastic nod in the affirmative. During the anaesthetic, everyone from the practice came to have a look. Our head nurse Kelly, missing her lunch and staying past her usual finishing time, could not stop grinning as she handled the most unusual patient of the year, expertly maintaining the anaesthesia. Even Sue from reception came to have a look. She hates snakes but loves dogs and cats and is fascinated by flamboyant birds.

Moments later, the X-rays confirmed there were no obvious hereditary issues. The blood samples will take a few days to be analysed. More than ever, we await them with baited breath. Vinnie's future as a breeding vulture hangs in the balance like, on a good day, he hangs in the air. And so does the rest of his species.

Flower Farm and Happy Farm

Nestling on the banks of the river Swale and off the beaten track, Catton is not somewhere you really pass through. My first association with the village was as a new vet in Thirsk. The job of attending to the rescue dogs at the Jerry Green Rescue Centre mainly fell to me and I visited every two weeks to vaccinate and health-check the miscellany of canines there. I became friendly with Chris and Hillary who were the custodians. Their enthusiasm was infectious and I loved my visits, although, as I spent most of the time kneeling on the kennel floors, my trousers took on an interesting odour, the most fragrant component of which was Jeyes Fluid. The smell evoked memories of helping with my grandparents' boarding kennels when I was a small boy.

I also spent plenty of time at the farm on the way into the village. The impressive Simmental cattle there thrived on the rich riverside grass. One night, I was called to calve a cow. She was trying to deliver twins and two water bags had appeared at the same time. The squashed space gave one of them the appearance of an elongated party balloon, causing both bafflement and alarm to the farmer, who called me in to help.

But it has been a while since I've visited Catton twice in two weeks. The first was to catch up with an old friend called Sahra. Three of her alpacas were thin and it was a question of solving the problem; an examination and then, crucially, a faeces test to check for worms was required. Afterwards, she showed me her new venture, which was farming of a totally different kind but went hand-in-hand alongside her animals. Sahra had branched out into flower farming! The outdoor beds were bursting with cornflowers of all colours and were peaceful, apart from the noise of the bees and birds.

"I pick up the alpaca poo, mix it with water and make a liquid called 'alpaca poo tea'. I use it to fertilize my flowers," Sahra explained. Inside a polytunnel, there was another example of sustainability in action. Sheep fleece was used as a slug repellent (its strands are barbed and rough under a slug's tummy) and alpaca fleece was used as a weed suppressant. It was a cornucopia of colours and scents with roses, sweet peas, peonies and sweet william, all powered by the fertile alpaca faeces. I picked a bunch for Anne.

Down the road, there was more sustainable diversity to be found. The Catton Kitchen grows its own vegetables and salad leaves for sale in vegetable boxes. Eggs from their hens go into each box too and Amy, the owner, planter and chief weeder, explained that "these were laid this morning. Most eggs people buy from shops are already two weeks old."

I had been called to see a couple of stubbornly lame sheep, which were simple to treat. Once done, I had a tour of the gardens. The hens and pigs are fed on the excess produce from the garden, so nothing is wasted. The veg box I had ordered was nearly ready for collection, but not before I'd picked the final salad leaves and even harvested my own cauliflower. The farm has its own chef and hosts parties where the homegrown produce is used for *al fresco* meals. It was certainly small scale and not a way of feeding the masses, but that wasn't the point. I quizzed Amy about the economics: did it pay? There was some vigorous nodding. "By year two we were making a profit," she said.

Later that evening, I was in the good books: for Anne a beautiful bunch of fresh, English flowers and the most delicious cauli for tea!

Henley Royal Regatta

Anne and I had a week off recently. It was a break that had been months in the planning, but was fraught with potential pitfalls, most of which were out of our control. The first came when we called to book the campervan into a campsite for three days. "I'm afraid you have to book the whole week," was the friendly but insistent reply.

And that was the start of our week at Henley Royal Regatta. The campsite was directly across the river from the action and a few minutes' walk from the finishing straight, although to be fair, the whole two-kilometre course was pretty straight. We hadn't been before, so it was a step into the unknown. Both Jack and Archie were hoping to race – Jack for university and Archie for school. Both were optimistic (they take after me) but the competition was tough to the point of being international, and Archie's crew missed out on a place by a devastatingly close two seconds. Fortunately for our holiday plans, Jack's boat got through.

Booking the camping was just the first challenge for the non-rowers. What followed was a detailed analysis of dress codes and the qualifications for entry into each of the enclosures. Anne needed a new dress (which was lovely) and I, apparently, needed a new hat. A panama hat. The day before we left Yorkshire, I called into Humphrey and Tilly's in Thirsk and uttered words I never thought I'd hear issuing from my mouth.

"I'd like to buy a panama hat, please." Not one of the staff laughed or even smirked. They are very professional in that shop.

"The black band around the hat dates back to the death of Queen Victoria, when workers on the Panama Canal were required to wear something black," explained the tailor. "Of course, they all wore these hats to keep the sun off their heads and that is why they look like this."

Equipped with new accoutrements and the van, we arrived in reasonable style.

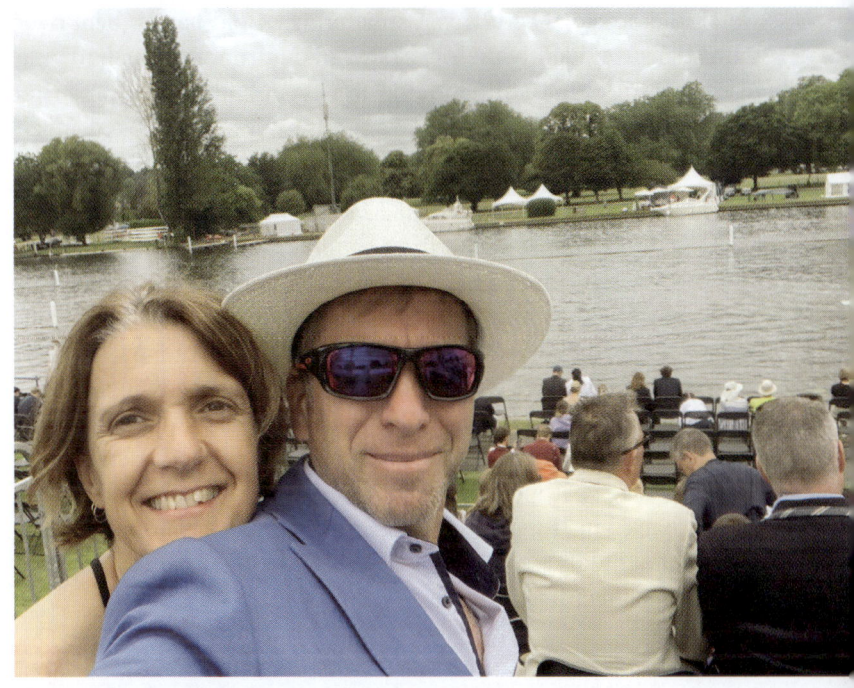

Anne and I enjoying a very different experience at Henley Royal Regatta, watching our boys race.

Henley Royal Regatta is like Wimbledon for rowing. There were fewer strawberries, but just as much Pimm's. It quickly became clear that it genuinely was the home for the world's elite rowers. Pursuing each race down the course was an elegant wooden boat with the umpire standing at the bow like Leonardo DiCaprio in *Titanic*, although clutching a flag to wave in case of infringement rather than Rose. One of the umpires was one of the world's most amazing athletes, Sir Matthew Pinsent. And other Olympic winners and world record holders were around too, so it was a privilege to watch them race. There was a smattering of old hands, bent over with sticks – evidently their backs worn out from too much rowing in earlier life – but still enjoying the event and dressed in stripy club blazers. Amongst the glad rags, my new hat looked much more at home than it had been in Thirsk the day before.

The first race of the afternoon had Jack in action, in the Bath crew. They were up against a boat from Denmark, although it turned out only two were Danish. One was American and the other Swiss. It was a close call, but despite inappropriately loud cheering from Anne and me, they were knocked out in the first round. Afterwards, we went to commiserate at the tented boathouse where hundreds of boats were residing, expecting to find four upset scullers. But not so. We watched from a distance; the four vanquished friends were laughing and chatting with their adversaries, patting each other on the back and forging new friendships. Old-fashioned as this event undoubtedly is, it was lovely to see that the best traditions of sportsmanship still pervaded.

Polish Thesis, Wittgenstein and Dogs in Prams

Perusing the practices' emails is always interesting. After a day away, catching up with the goings-on with Anne from the comfort of the sofa, with a glass of wine late one evening, she said, "Have you seen the email from the Polish vet?"

I hadn't, but Anne explained: "He's a vet but also studying English and has written his thesis about one of your books." I was intrigued and immediately opened the emails to have a read.

"Dear Dr Norton," it began, politely. "I have been practising as a pig vet in Poland for ten years. My other passion is English and I joined a local university to study as an extramural pupil. Attached is my thesis for my BA, which is based on translation of two chapters from your book, regards Piotr."

I read on. Piotr's thesis was arranged into three sections: the translation process, influential translators across history and their techniques, and the translations themselves (of the chapters 'Foot and Mouth Disease: A Return to the Dark Ages' and 'Things Stuck in Animals and Animals Stuck in Things'). At the end there were some additional translator's notes. It reminded me of the time I discovered, from a Polish friend, that our TV programme *The Yorkshire Vet* was being shown in Poland. Of course, not many people know about Yorkshire in Poland, so the name had been changed to *The Vet with a Heart*. The new moniker made me smile. Also, the time when I received, out of the blue, a copy of a translation of my first book into Slovakian! The copy still sits, largely unread, in a bookcase somewhere upstairs.

Piotr's thesis turned out to be a work of genius and far superior to the original chapters. The first section discussed the various techniques used by different translators. Roman Jakobson, a Russo-American linguist with his tripartite division theory of translation, lends a quote to open the thesis: "Languages differ essentially in what they *must* convey and not what they *may* convey." I looked forward to what Piotr would make of the section about the heifer who got stuck on a tiny bridge and was hoisted into the air by a large digger. Of course, I had no idea whether his translation was accurate, but the detail and depth of interrogation of my text in his final conclusion told me it must have been precise.

One fascinating section referenced the challenges with translation of cultural topics, historical events or sporting stories. In one part of the book I had compared the odd animal antics to a narrative in a Mr Men book. The joke must surely have been lost in Polish, so too a couple of references to the game of cricket. Perhaps my biggest *faux pas* (but one I could never have expected to be a *faux pas* at the time of writing) was my preamble to the inaction of the Ministry of Agriculture, Fisheries and Food at the start of the Foot and Mouth Disease outbreak in 2001. I drew comparisons with the "Phoney War", where similar inactivity occurred shortly after Britain declared war on Germany in 1939 following the latter's invasion of Piotr's homeland. With bigger things to worry about at that time, the Polish obviously were totally unaware of this phrase, rendering it practically impossible to translate. Even Jakobsson would have been scratching his head.

After finishing the bulk of Piotr's masterpiece, I flicked through the other emails which had escaped my attention. A second opinion from Noel Fitzpatrick had agreed with my initial assessment (phew). And there was another email, addressed to a colleague, entitled "dogs in prams" which contained a large selection of photos of, you guessed it, dogs in prams. It provided the perfect antidote to the heavy content of the earlier ones: "As requested, dogs in prams. Take your pick."

Alpacas

I've been seeing plenty of alpacas recently. For better or worse, I don't often get chance to don my wellies and waterproof trousers on the farm these days. But trips to see alpacas and other pet farm animals puts a smile on my face more than it disrupts my day in the clinic.

There are not too many vets who jump at the chance to see a camelid. Once, nobody really knew anything about these curious creatures from South America. Were they fluffy ponies or sheep with long legs? And what about the spitting? No vets or farmers had experienced this behaviour when alpacas arrived in Yorkshire twenty-five years ago. But now, smallholders, vets and farmers are more accustomed to these novel creatures.

The main and routine job is castration. Males like to live in groups, but their natural tendencies are very driven by hormones. Their urge to mate, scrap, fight and even bite each other in the gonads is strong. Neutering solves this problem and evens out any bad tempers.

My most recent job was also all about the hormones. Although, to call it a job was stretching the truth somewhat. My role was to introduce two friends and four alpacas. Ian has a mobile farm, taking his animals to schools and educating children about their ways. He wanted babies

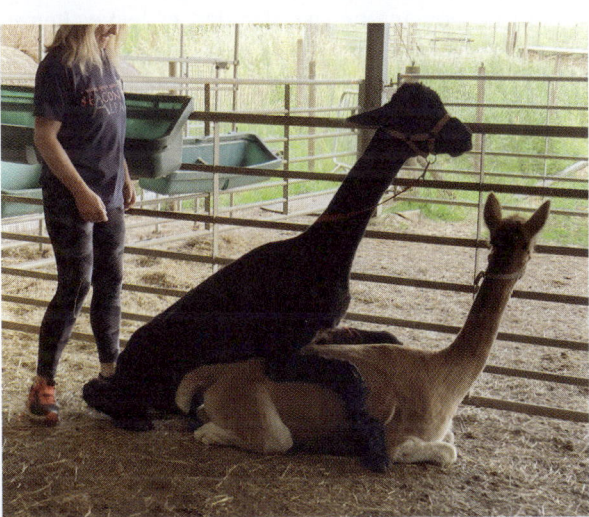

The supervised mating alpacas is an important job for an alpaca farmer like Jackie. It's very different to the way most animals mate!

(called cria) from two of his female alpacas. As he explained his plan, I had an idea. Another friend, Jackie, has an alpaca farm and a thriving business both breeding cria and taking visitors on alpaca treks. I made a few phone calls and a date was made.

A few weeks later, on a warm sunny afternoon, I sucked on an ice pop at Jackie's as we awaited the arrival of Ian and his females. I'd seen alpacas mating before and it's a very interesting experience – different to most animals on the farm. The boys – Red and Indiana Jones – were already looking forward to their afternoon encounter. Indiana Jones, with bouffant hair and fluffy ears, looked like he'd been preening himself in front of the mirror for most of the day. If he had, it would have been wasted time because both females (Belinda and Humbug) were delighted to see them no matter what they looked like. There was a huge amount of high-pitched chirping, then both females immediately sat down on the floor; Humbug on a comfy bed of deep hay. Alpacas mate lying down and Red and Indi wasted no time positioning themselves on top.

The process takes up to an hour (!) and is a gentle scene of contentment. There is no commotion, no urgency and no vigorous thrusting. During the mating, Red even appeared to lean in and kiss Belinda on her neck and caress her with his front legs. There was little requirement for supervision, although after it is finished it's important to make sure the boys don't start fighting. Not wishing to be voyeuristic, we decided to leave them to it and retired for a cup of tea. Ian and Jackie related stories of the challenges and successes of their versions of farming diversification. I have to say, it is heart-warming to see how it *is* very possible to carve a life with animals in a non-conventional fashion.

We finished our tea just as a group of about fifteen alpaca trekkers returned. They all had smiles on their faces and had clearly enjoyed the relaxing walk. They'd be back for more. Meanwhile, in the barn, Red, Belinda, Indiana Jones and Humbug were still at it. I couldn't hang around. Evening surgery beckoned and I couldn't be late. My excuse would have been too weird: "Sorry I'm late, I've been watching four alpacas mating."

Acknowledgements

As ever, there is a multitude of people to thank for my latest culmination of collected stories. All the editors at *The Yorkshire Post* have provided constant support for my weekly column. This has been the stimulus for all of the "diary" series of books, published by local publisher Great Northern Books. On a regular basis, clients comment on my weekly musings and it is a pleasure to bring the stories to a wider audience.

This book would have a different title were it not for the inception of Thirsk Veterinary Centre. Being part of the growth of this nascent business has been a wonderful experience, as has reconnecting with the animal-owning public of the town where I live, not to mention some of the pets I have known for many years. This venture would have been considerably more difficult without the hard work and dedication of Anne and Isabella.

The production team of *The Yorkshire Vet* have been near constant companions over the last ten years, helping guide me through the weird world of television. It was through them that I made a hesitant phone call to Lucy Pittaway, whose amazing portrait of my lovely Jack Russell, Emmy, adorns the waiting room at our practice and is also on the front cover of this book. It can be purchased, I think, from her galleries all over the north of the country, along with her other majestic paintings. I'm so grateful for everyone who has helped bring this book together, especially my editor Ross Jamieson and creative director David Burrill.

Also by Julian:

Horses, Heifers and Hairy Pigs: The Life of a Yorkshire Vet

A Yorkshire Vet Through the Seasons

The Diary of a Yorkshire Vet

On Call with a Yorkshire Vet

A Yorkshire Vet: The Next Chapter

All Creatures: Heart-warming Tales from a Yorkshire Vet

*Adventures with a Yorkshire Vet:
Lambing Time and Other Animal Tales*

*Adventures with a Yorkshire Vet:
The Lucky Foal and Other Animal Tales*

Ruminations of a Yorkshire Vet

New Pastures for a Yorkshire Vet

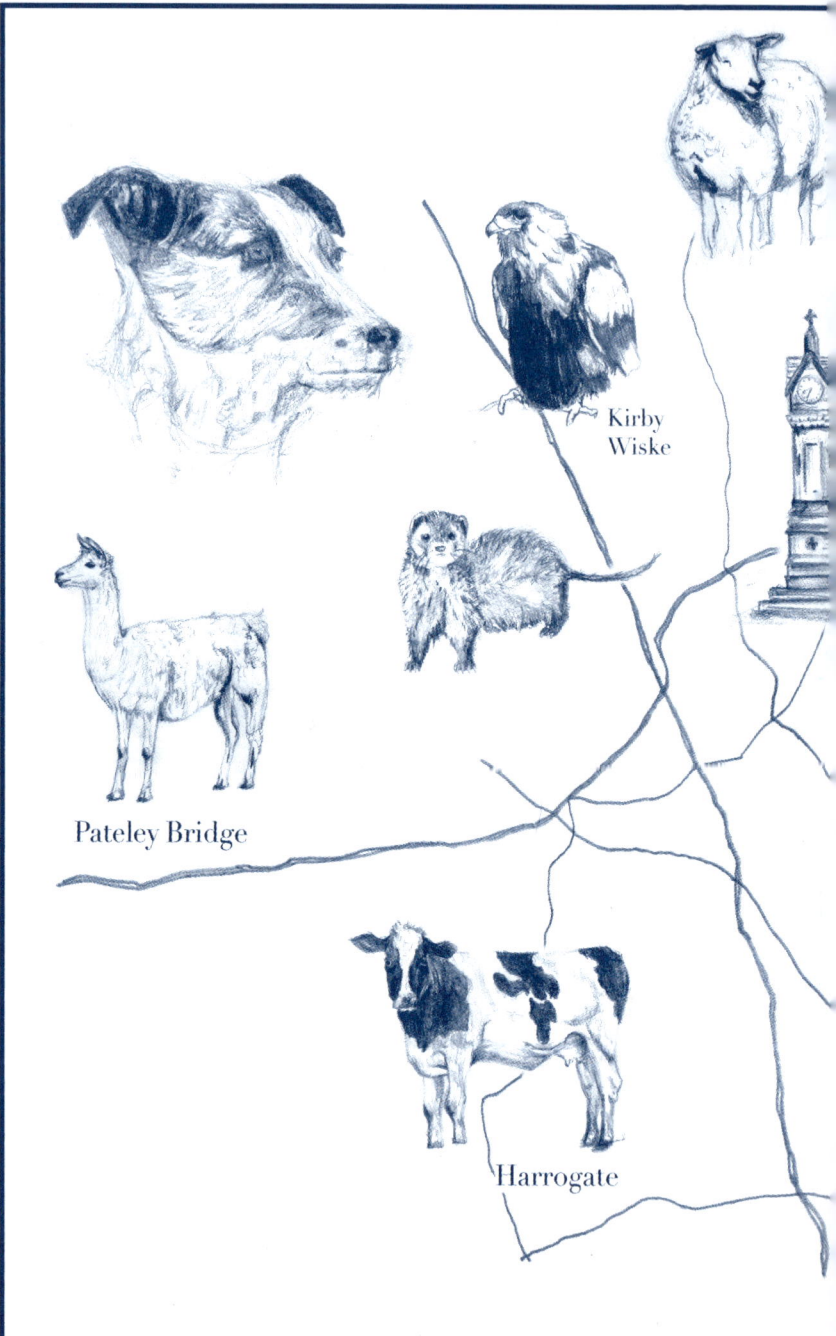